BIG PICTURE THINKING

Using Central Coherence Theory
to Support Social Skills

A Book for Students

Aileen Zeitz Collucci, MA, CCC

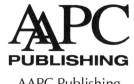

AAPC Publishing

AAPC Publishing
6448 Vista Dr.
Shawnee, KS 66218
www.aapcpublishing.net

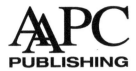

© 2011 AAPC Publishing
6448 Vista Dr.
Shawnee, KS 66218
www.aapcpublishing.net

Publisher's Cataloging-in-Publication

Collucci, Aileen Zeitz.

Big picture thinking : using central coherence theory to support social skills : a book for students / Aileen Zeitz Collucci. -- Shawnee Mission, Kan. : AAPC Pub., c2011.

p. ; cm.

ISBN: 978-1-934575-86-4
LCCN: 2011934185
Includes bibliographical references.
Audience: parents, teachers and students.
Summary: A series of lessons and information for teaching students to analyze social situations, break them down into their component parts and then adding everything together again to create a whole-- the big picture.

1. Autistic children--Behavior modification--Study and teaching.
2. Autistic youth--Behavior modification--Study and teaching.
3. Social skills in children--Study and teaching. 4. Social skills in adolescence--Study and teaching. 5. Social interaction in children--Study and teaching. 6. Social interaction in adolescence--Study and teaching. 7. Social participation--Study and teaching.
8. Interpersonal relations in children--Study and teaching.
9. Interpersonal relations in adolescence--Study and teaching.
10. [Social skills. 11. Interpersonal relations.] I. Title.

RJ506.A9 C655 2011
618.92/85882--dc23   1108

This book is designed in Optima. Interior and cover photos: ©2011 Photos.com

Printed in the United States of America.

Dedication

For Daddy.

I miss you more than words can say.

Table of Contents

Acknowledgments

My relationship with this book has been very similar to the relationships I have had with many of the children that I work with. In the beginning, the book was like a lot of my students are when I first start working with them, kind of inconspicuous, yet totally noticeable at the same time. It was smart and said a lot of important things, but it was a little disorganized and sometimes confusing even to me. It needed some tending to, like a garden, and it began to blossom just a little bit more every time I went back to it to help it grow. Once it did develop, it surprised me how beautiful and brilliant it really was. It became more than I ever expected. I hope it will continue to surprise me and exceed my expectations, just as so many of my students have.

There are many people I would like to thank for their help and support as I worked on this book. First, I would like to thank Kirsten McBride from AAPC, a wonderful and extremely talented editor, who saw the importance of this book and guided me expertly toward perfecting it into a "cohesive" useful tool. Her expertise in editing and her background knowledge about autism spectrum disorders is an awesome combination. Thank you to my early reviewers, Dr. Margaret Meth, director of William Paterson University's Communication Disorders Clinic, AAPC authors Kari Dunn Buron and Sue Diamond, and Allyson Castelli, special education teacher, Paterson Public Schools.

It has been most rewarding for me that so many of my Social Skills Group clients and their families are still in touch with me after many years. Too many to mention, but you know who you are, and I thank you greatly for believing in the process and in my abilities. An extra-special thank-you goes out to Diana Cicchino and her son, Marco Antonio Cicchino, for trusting me with so much. The work we have done together has been rewarding in so many ways, and without a doubt it has contributed to this book as well.

I have many supportive friends and colleagues. Many I see on a regular basis, and some I don't see often because they live far away. I know everyone in my life has lent their support in one way or another, and although I would like to name every one of you, that would be challenging. Look carefully through the book because I may have acknowledged you somewhere.

Specifically, I would like to thank the following people, Nicole Mitarotonda, for her amazing psychological consultations; Faith Bell, for her rave review, her creative contributions to the cover of this book, her beautiful photographs, and for listening to me complaining.

I would like to make one more very special mention of a very special friend, Serenity Marie Dolan, the most beautiful angel in heaven. I think of you every day. Further, to my closest friends, really my extended family, who listened to and learned from me whether they felt like it or not, and all of their children who have unknowingly served as "research subjects" at one time or another, Michele Kaplan, Melissa Siegel, Meryl and Michael Budnick and "kids": Emily, Avery, Rebecca, Hayley and Marisa the Great.

A huge thank-you goes out to my "second mother," Sandy Collucci. You are a wonderful grandmother to my son and a fabulous "personal assistant" and laundry fairy to me. Without your help in so many areas, I don't think I would have been able to complete this project. Thank you for being my friend.

Another huge thank-you goes to my mother, Susan Zeitz, for all of her expert proofreading and suggestions. It is duly noted that without your contributions, I probably would not have known what to do with this manuscript in the first place. Thank you for being my mom and friend even when it's been difficult. Evan, Susan, and Samantha Zeitz, miles are meaningless, and I love you all more than words can say. Some day I hope we will have the freedom to see each other much more frequently.

Last, but never least, to my boy, Cary Alexander Collucci. It is with great pleasure that I tell you this … I'm finally, really and truly, done with the book, so I will be more than happy to play with you. You are my life, beautiful boy. I love you.

Central Coherence Theory and Big Picture Thinking:
An Introduction for Parents and Educators

Learning how to deal with social situations is a lifelong task. As children grow and develop, they continue to encounter new social challenges, in increasingly complex contexts. A preschooler needs to navigate and master simple things like sharing a toy, whereas school-age children have to negotiate more complicated things like "sharing" friends. High-school students need to have insight into which of their friends they trust enough to share their science notes with, or which of their friends they trust enough to share personal secrets with. As adults in work environments, we need to be able to work cooperatively and support our coworkers while simultaneously accommodating the needs of our boss, our boss's bosses, and so on.

Being able to negotiate social interactions successfully is a life skill essential for future success. Without this ability, one will have considerable difficulty getting along with others, forging friendships, finding and keeping a job, and much more. For example, learning to drive a car and being a safe motorist requires essential attention, prediction and perspective taking skills, not to mention many other abilities that are social and interactional in nature.

Central Coherence Theory: "Big Picture Thinking"

Interpreting social situations requires first an understanding of the context, or the "whole" of a situation, as it is happening. One must then be able to "add" all of the parts together and arrive at a "sum total" quickly and effortlessly. If we are limited in our ability to make sense of the main idea of what is happening around us, our social interactions will be less fluid than those of our peers, and this can make it difficult to participate in the give-and-take of everyday situations.

Many people who have difficulties with social cognition, including those on the autism spectrum, are not able to see the Big Picture of a situation, described in the literature as a weakness in central coherence (Frith, 1989). That is, they tend to focus, or even "hyper-focus," on the details within the larger whole of a concept, conversation, story, picture or situation, and, therefore, have difficulty recognizing the main idea. In his work *The Extreme Male-Brain Theory of Autism*, Simon Baron-Cohen (1999) states that while central coherence is difficult to define, "The essence of it is the normal drive to integrate information into a context, or 'Gestalt'" (p. 17).

Statistics show that boys are 4 times as likely as girls to develop autism and 10 times more likely to be diagnosed with Asperger Syndrome (Goleman, 2006a). Baron-Cohen (1999) describes the neurological profiles of people with these disorders as "an extreme form of the male brain" (pp. 35-36). He relates that this "extreme" male brain is not well equipped for emotional empathy, but it has intellectual strengths such as understanding systems like the "stock market, computer software and quantum physics." In contrast, the "extreme female brain excels at empathy and understanding others' thoughts and feelings," which fits very nicely into professions like teaching and counseling. They have more difficulties with "systems," such as applying directions when driving (Baron-Cohen, p. 34; Goleman, p. 139).

Baron-Cohen's discussion directs us to understand important differences in processing styles and how tasks related to recognizing information that is best processed as a whole, such as understanding the emotional states of others, have a neurological basis. The "polar opposites" of men vs. women are highlighted, but we know that a spectrum of abilities in processing style is possible. In general, most people fall somewhere in the middle of that spectrum, not to mention that many women are gifted with systematizing and many men are brilliant at showing empathy (Goleman, 2006a).

> ... we cannot lump together all people who have strengths in understanding details as having a weakness.

Related to teaching social skills, what is most salient here is that the ideas of Baron-Cohen and others remind us that we cannot lump together all people who have strengths in understanding details as having a weakness. It also helps us recognize the differences between males and females. Those experienced in working with girls on the autism spectrum are well aware that they are more challenging to diagnose and treat, mainly because they don't "look" as strikingly impaired or fit the same "model" of symptomology as boys.

Most important, the findings of Baron-Cohen and others give us a solid beginning point for assessment and intervention. We can examine a client's processing style and determine if there is a weakness in gestalt thinking that needs to be accommodated or supported to help the person recognize social information in context. Having a balanced brain, where both holistic thinking and more analytical thought processes are present, is an important goal. We know from the growing research on neuroplasticity, for example, that if we provide the brain with appropriate experiences highlighting a more effective processing style, we will be able to help the brain habituate to that processing style (Schwartz & Begley, 2002).

Identifying Students With Weaknesses in Central Coherence: Can They See the Forest for the Trees?

Several writers (Baron-Cohen, 1999; Wieder & Greenspan, 2005; Winner, 2006) have suggested that part of being successful with social cognition is related to having effective information-processing skills that focus on the whole rather than the sum of its parts. How then might we identify such thinking patterns in an individual so we can effectively support him or her in being more successful in the social realm? What does this processing style look like in individuals who have social-cognitive deficits?

As mentioned, sometimes clients are too focused on individual details and, therefore, have difficulty "getting to the point" in a conversation. At other times, they are only concerned about their own thoughts. Or maybe they are overly attentive to sticking to the rules, not only on their own behalf but also by acting as the "rule police" for others. In doing so, they not only annoy and alienate peers but are missing out on the fun of a game or experience with friends.

A great example is the student who is asked to talk about a specific event, such as a trip he took with his family. Rather than giving a brief overview of the highlights, many students with social-cognitive deficits respond by giving a lengthy monologue that includes every single detail about the trip and never gets to the main idea. It might look a little bit like this:

Teacher: So how was your spring break vacation to Mexico?

Student: Well, first we woke up at 6 a.m. and finished packing our clothes. Then we ate breakfast. I had pancakes because it was Saturday. I always have pancakes on Saturday mornings. After that, we put our luggage in the car. My mom packed my clothes for me, but I also brought a book, my Nintendo, and three games to play. Then we got in the car and drove down the Garden State Parkway to get to Newark Liberty International Airport, where we parked the car in the long-term parking lot because we were going to be gone for 10 days. We walked for a little more than 5 minutes to get to the entrance to Continental Airlines. Then we had to check in our suitcases and show the lady behind the counter our tickets. Then we looked at the departure screen to find out what gate we needed to go to. Then we went through the security thing and boy was I mad. I had to take off my shoes. And those security officials looked so mean …

So far, there is a lot of "answer" but almost no information about what the listener was **really** interested in hearing about: the trip as a whole. It is important to note that from the child's perspective, he is responding appropriately, because that's how the memories have been stored in his brain.

Now, consider the conversational partner in this instance. Her feelings and comfort level with the discourse situation, as well as her feelings about the communication skills of the other person, will most certainly be affected.

I currently work with an 18-year-old young man with a diagnosis of high-functioning autism who loves watching the show "America's Next Top Model." Of course, this didn't totally surprise me since he is an 18-year-old male, and the show features beautiful young women. Nevertheless, it was not a typical choice. I told him I had never seen the show and wasn't sure what it was about. I asked him to tell me about it, and he was more than happy to elaborate on his interest.

> ... sometimes clients are too focused on individual details and, therefore, have difficulty "getting to the point" in a conversation.

He began to explain the episodes and tell me about who was currently on the show, using the show's jargon and specifics that I couldn't follow. When I started asking clarifying questions, he decided it would be easier for us to look it up in Wikipedia "where he could show me what he was talking about." I actually thought this was a brilliant idea since all I knew was that the host was Tyra Banks and that at the end of the season someone probably becomes a fashion model.

I expected that he would start at the top of the Wikipedia entry, as I would have, and that we would read through it together so that at the end, I would have a better idea about how the episodes worked. But I had forgotten that I frequently arrive at unexpected places with my students. In this case, the student scrolled down through the entry and clicked on one of the charts that listed every season (called "cycles" on this program) of the show, 1 through 15. He moved right to the spot in the chart labeled Cycle 14. "We are in cycle 15 now, but I will show you cycle 14," he explained. One more click, and we were on a new page, where he scrolled quickly down to another chart that listed the vital statistics of all of the contestants featured in that season. Then he proceeded to read the list out loud to me.

Sitting there next to him and listening, it occurred to me to ask the question, "What is it about this show that you like so much? Are you interested in modeling, fashion or photography?" "No," he replied, "I just like the 'call-out' order (how the models are eliminated) and the 'destinations' that the finalists get to go to." Then he proceeded to recite, from memory, each and every cycle of the show and which destination was featured. This was exhausting for me, but enjoyable for him. Not to mention that it was very hard to bring him back into the reciprocal nature of true conversation.

We generally tell children in need of "social" help, particularly those who need to work on expanding their social circles, that a good way to make new friends is to find people with common interests. Asking about "favorites" is a way to start to determine if you have a similar interest to someone else. You can get to know someone by asking questions like, "What's your favorite TV show?" and see if you have that in common. However, the example above shows that a "favorite" can be a favorite for an entirely different reason to someone who has difficulty with holistic processing and storing memories in an episodic fashion. Imagine my 18-year-old client attempting to engage a peer about his favorite TV show. Most certainly, it would be difficult for him and the peer to move any further than simply finding out that they both liked the same show. Having a conversation, enjoying the show together, or delving further into interests around the show would be difficult, especially if engaging with a neurotypical peer.

If you take a minute and think about the clients, students, or children that you work or live with, you will probably recognize some of these other examples:

- They frequently become over-focused on their own thoughts or ideas.

- They are easily distracted by a small detail that appears inconsequential to others but gigantic to them.

- They have difficulty moving on from challenging moments with peers, and they might even hold "grudges."

- They have a hard time engaging in conversations with others and always seem to be "off topic;" however, they are great at practicing "staying on the topic" during a structured lesson.

- They are constantly hyper-aware of rules and abide by them completely. They also act as a rule enforcer with their peers or even with adults.

- They remember specifics about past events that are sometimes even more specific than necessary, like what day and time it was when you last played a particular game.

- They have difficulty with reading comprehension and tasks that require understanding the main idea of what they are reading. They are "early readers," or fluent readers because of excellent decoding skills, but they have a lot of trouble understanding what they have read. Making mistakes with reading homonyms is common, reading the sentence with the word "tear": "there was a tear in her eye" as "there was a tear in her dress" (Baron-Cohen, 1999, p. 17).

- They have difficulty giving directions or providing a verbal or written summary about something that they know a lot about.

- They may have difficulties with writing assignments in general.

- They confuse facts and opinions, when they are expressing themselves or when others are speaking to them.

- They often have difficulty making inferences, predictions or solving problems, as well as other critical thinking tasks, and abstractions like humor and figurative language. In many cases, they are unable to determine the meaning of certain idiomatic expressions, even when presented in context.

- They like to play or do the same things over and over again.

> They have difficulty with reading comprehension and tasks that require understanding the main idea of what they are reading.

Although this is not a complete list of *every* behavior, it clearly gives examples of weak central coherence, or the difficulty with gestalt thinking, that is typically observed in our clients. People with these types of information-processing difficulties do not always have cognitive deficits or challenges related to understanding the rules of social interactions, but they do exhibit a performance deficit. This means they can tell you exactly what you want to hear about doing things the "right" way, but they have difficulty enacting those rules in the moment. In school settings, these are the kids who are challenged by working in groups, cause interruptions in class discussions or lectures, and run out of time on projects and tests. Overall, they are generally isolated from others because their difficulties cause them to alienate friends or co-workers.

Becoming Connected

I have worked as a speech-language pathologist for more than 20 years. For the most part, I began to gain experience working with children with an autism spectrum disorder (ASD) while employed at a private special education school in New York City. At the time, autism was becoming a concern for many parents of young children, and professionals in the field were responding with research. Words like *spectrum, pervasive developmental disorder-NOS* and *Asperger Syndrome* were being introduced and entered into the fourth edition of the *Diagnostic and Statistical Manual of Mental Disorders* (American Psychiatric Association, 2000).

As professionals, we responded by utilizing these new descriptive terms to help educate parents. As speech-language pathologists, we focused on pragmatic language development and the precursory behaviors that are necessary to develop reciprocal communication, the one aspect that seemed to be the biggest challenge for our students.

In 1997 I became connected with another speech-language pathologist, who "recruited" me to do social skills groups with children in her private practice in New Jersey. She and a colleague had observed a need for social intervention with the "autistic" population, and they had responded by putting together a program of "co-treatment" groups that included both a speech-language pathologist and a mental health professional. When I joined the team, we offered four groups, but within a short time, word got around, and our numbers began growing. At the height of our program, we were running between 15 and 20 groups per week, with an average of about 6-8 children in each group.

Shortly after I began working there, I took responsibility for running the group program, creating intervention plans, working with parents, and leading groups. I became increasingly involved in researching methods and programs and adapting and implementing them into my lesson plans. I recognized that as the children were learning, I too was improving upon my understanding of social processes as they occurred in my own life. I read books, watched movies and television programs, and constantly observed in order to pick up on the "hidden curriculum" (Myles, Trautman, & Schelvan, 2004) that my students were missing.

The work I was doing developing the curriculum turned into a 24-hour-a-day job, much like learning social skills is a 24-hour-a-day job for those with social-cognitive deficits. In order for students to learn, they needed to constantly be thinking about social skills, not just "turning it on" once a week for an hour in group. Similarly, in order for me to be an effective clinician, I had to focus on thinking about social skills 24 hours a day.

Building an Effective Intervention Program Using Evidence-Based Practices

In addition to central coherence theory, theory of mind (Baron-Cohen, Leslie, & Frith, 1985) and executive dysfunction theory (McEvoy, Rogers, & Pennington, 1993) have been researched extensively as two other core deficit areas that may be present in individuals with social-cognitive deficits. While this book focuses on understanding and teaching gestalt thinking, the other areas of need should not be overlooked in intervention planning.

Some researchers have indicated that there is a continuum of ability with regard to central coherence, indicating that there are weaknesses at both "low" and "high" levels (Happé, 1999; Plaisted, Saksida, Alcantara, & Weisblatt, 2003). These students are exhibiting a weakness in their ability to "draw together or integrate individual pieces of information to establish meaning" (Plaisted et al., p. 375). In my experiences working with these types of clients, they are lacking in their ability to process the "whole" of an experience, or the overall context, which is necessary in order to integrate oneself into a social situation.

> **... a large part of a social learning curriculum should focus on helping students "see" how individual pieces of information fit into a larger context, so that they may begin to become more of a gestalt thinker, or "big picture thinker."**

Therefore, it makes sense that a large part of a social learning curriculum should focus on helping students "see" how individual pieces of information fit into a larger context, so that they may begin to become more of a gestalt thinker, or "big picture thinker." Skills may be broken down in order to get a student started thinking about behaviors. Then, these skills must be put back together again, into a manageable whole, in order for them to efficiently process the social situation. This book does just that – it highlights some important social processes and reinforces the importance of putting it all together – the long-term goal of a social learning curriculum.

In addition to the research of Frith on central coherence theory, this book and my intervention methods rest on the written work of many other professionals in the field of social-cognitive deficits. In no particular order, Mel Levine, Daniel Goleman, Simon Baron-Cohen, Uta Frith, Carol Gray, and Tony Attwood have all been influential. Their understanding of how to better support students on the spectrum has laid the groundwork for building a better curriculum. Each of these professionals has elaborated to some extent on the following points:

1. **People need to have good perspective taking abilities in order to be successful in their socialization efforts.** Referred to as theory of mind, frequently abbreviated as ToM (Baron-Cohen et al., 1985), this describes the ability to understand the thoughts and beliefs of another person. Such understanding and the ability to recognize others' intentions and points of view are critical aspects of socializing and communicating. That is, it permits us to monitor our responses and adjust our behaviors, as needed, during an interaction (Winner, 2006).

   The ability to successfully recognize what is happening in someone else's mind is referred to as "mindsight" by neuroscientists (Goleman, 2006a). This means people are able to use the contextual clues around them, such as facial expressions, tone of voice, or gestures, as well as other visual clues from the situation, such as where the interaction is taking place, to infer what the other person is thinking. Without mindsight, we are unable to engage with others in meaningful relationships, including displaying empathy. Mindsight is the understanding that others have thoughts and feelings that are different from our own. The ability to make inferences about what those thoughts and feelings are requires gestalt thinking.

In individuals with autism and similar disorders, weaknesses in perspective taking can vary in severity and must be assessed accordingly in order to formulate appropriate goals. Deficits in ToM run the gamut from what is called "mindblindness," or the complete inability to recognize the point of view of another person, to what Michelle Winner refers to as "impaired interactive perspective taking" (Winner, 2007a, p. 9). The latter term describes individuals who are not "mindblind" but have weaknesses in perspective taking.

> **Goals for social learning should reflect the importance of understanding the perspective of others and how their thoughts, feelings, and interests differ from our own.**

2. **Emotional relatedness is at the core of interpersonal interactions and is necessary for truly meaningful connections with others.** Many people with social difficulties display weaknesses in their ability to connect emotions to experiences and then store memories of such events in a holistic manner. It has been shown that the emotional significance of an event has an effect on our memory of the event (Kensinger, 2004) and that we are more likely to remember personal experiences that contain some emotional relevance for us (Conway et al., 1994). It has also been shown that emotions have an effect on attention to details. Our emotions affect our attention processes, whereby we are more apt to have the capacity to attend to the emotional arousal we feel and have less attentional resources available for information processing. Consequently, information central to the source of the emotion is stored in memory and the peripheral details less so (Easterbrook, 1959; Kensinger). In other words, we remember the "feeling" we attach to a past experience as a whole and then uncover more detailed information as we start to think more about it. This is typically the way most people store and retrieve their personal experiences. It is also a more socially acceptable way to relate such memories to other people, by giving a main idea statement first and then waiting to see if the person we are speaking with is available and interested before we divulge further details. As the conversation moves forward, and the discourse partner asks more questions, we begin revealing even more details, possibly even peripheral information that we may not have recalled initially.

Episodic memory is the storage of personal events. This includes the where and when and other context-relevant information and their associated emotions. The example earlier in this chapter where the student talks about his family vacation does not reveal any emotions that he may have connected to being with his family, having a new experience, or his enjoyment of it. Instead, we see a listing of temporal events that would be better titled "How to Take a Vacation."

Procedural memory refers to the long-term storage of how to do things like tie our shoes or drive a car. It helps us remember step-by-step directions about the cognitive and motor skills we need to complete such tasks. It often does not even require us to have conscious control or attention during retrieval. Our vacation student appears to store his personal experiences in a procedural manner, and, therefore, his explanations are exactly that. In addition to weaknesses in central coherence, weaknesses in emotional connectedness to people and experiences, and in overall emotional understanding, impact our ability to store memories in an episodic fashion. Engaging relationships and a solid understanding of our own emotions and those of the people around us are important aspects of social interactions. Highlighting how experiences are stored related to emotions is also essential when teaching social skills.

> *Goals for social learning should reflect emotional understanding and encourage, as naturalistically as possible, the enjoyment of simply having relationships with others and connecting memories to emotions and people.*

3. **Communicative competence is a large part of successful social interactions.**

   Communicative competence refers to how we use our language skills to verbally interact with others. It involves a person's **pragmatic knowledge** and the awareness of when to use particular types of linguistic constructions (Phelps-Terasaki & Phelps-Gunn, 2007). More specifically, pragmatic knowledge refers to comprehension of the social conventions of communication, such as turn-taking and staying on the topic. Being aware of when to use certain linguistic constructions allows us to use language for different social purposes. Examples of communicative competence include things like being able to produce an interrogative statement or question at an appropriate time in a conversation in order to gain information or being able to construct a narrative in an organized way to tell a listener about a personal experience.

   Communicative competence includes understanding the following contexts within an interaction:

   - **Situational context** – refers to the **physical environment** and the **audience** involved in the interaction. Where is the interaction taking place, and who is present? People use different types of linguistic constructions and rules based on these things. For example, we speak differently to someone we don't know very well versus a close friend, and a student speaks differently to a teacher versus a peer. We also speak differently when we are in the library versus in the gym.

   - **Discourse context** – refers to the functions of the language used and how effective it is for conveying a particular intent. This includes ***topics*** of conversation and management of the topic(s), as well as ***purpose***, which refers to the goals of the conversation and the type of linguistic structures that are utilized to achieve those goals. For example, recognizing that there are different reasons for communicating with others. Are we trying to get information or share our thoughts and feelings? Are we interviewing someone or engaging in a shared conversation? Are the topics that we are referring to appropriate for the audience and situation?

- **Semantic context** – refers to the meaning of a discourse interaction and certain aspects of language that can convey concepts or ideas. This includes **visual-gestural cues** (nonverbal aspects of communication), **abstractions** (communication of symbolic forms that are not direct), such as metaphors and figurative language and humor, and **pragmatic evaluation** (a speaker's ability to self-monitor his or her pragmatic skills throughout an interaction).

> ... pragmatic knowledge refers to comprehension of the social conventions of communication, such as turn-taking and staying on the topic.

Many children in need of support in the social arena have what might be considered age-appropriate language skills, yet they are not able to use these skills to complete the full range of social functions. Many are children who are frequently overlooked by educators and professionals, sometimes even speech-language pathologists, because "they talk so much" when, in reality, their talking is not always directly connected to the discourse situation around them. They have difficulty with initiating with others, taking turns, or monitoring the timing of their verbal contributions. Or they have challenges with simply using language for different purposes.

Additionally, some children have true linguistic deficits that impact on their pragmatic (social) language abilities. In other words, their challenges with expressive and receptive language is a large part of what causes problems for them in the social aspects of communication.

The true weakness is not in the amount of language that is produced; instead, it is the *interaction* between expressive language form, content, and use. **Form** refers to the shape and sound of the basic units of language and their combinations such as word endings, words, or sentence structure. **Content** refers to what individuals talk about or understand. Finally, the **Use** of language refers to why an individual is speaking and the ways in which he constructs conversations, depending upon what he knows about the listener and the context (Lahey, 1988). A breakdown in one area has an effect on the others. If somebody is not able to use the correct sentence structure, he probably won't be able to communicate his intent, or what he means to say, to someone else. Or, if a person is limited in the types of things he wants to say or talk about, he probably won't be able to engage effectively in conversation with others. The figure below exemplifies how these three areas of expressive language interact.

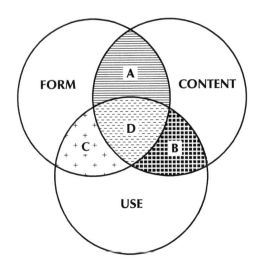

From *Language Disorders and Language Development* (p. 18) by Margaret Lahey, 1988, Boston, MA: Allyn & Bacon. Used with permission.

> *Goals for social learning should target communication skills, including knowing and understanding the "rules" of conversational interactions and being competent enough with language to communicate intentions appropriately.*

In the social skills groups that I work with, I illustrate all three of these areas: perspective taking, emotional relatedness, and communicative competence. I also emphasize the significant interrelationships among them. For example, weaknesses in perspective taking have an impact on communicative competence. If we don't understand what others are thinking, we might not give enough information to a listener when conversing. Furthermore, we won't be able to self-monitor communication breakdowns and make repairs as necessary. Or, if we have a limited ability to understand our own emotions in a situation, this will clearly affect how we understand the emotions of others.

In addition to those three points, I attempt to highlight the importance of self-awareness. I provide support for students and clients as they examine questions about themselves such as …

- What is your learning profile?
- How do you self-regulate?
- What are your stressors?
- What are your strengths?
- What are your weaknesses?
- What motivates you?
- What are your goals?

Understanding oneself solidifies work in the area of perspective taking, and it contributes greatly to progress in many other social areas. It also helps one to become a more successful self-advocate. Self-advocacy is an important aspect of achieving independence and success as an adult.

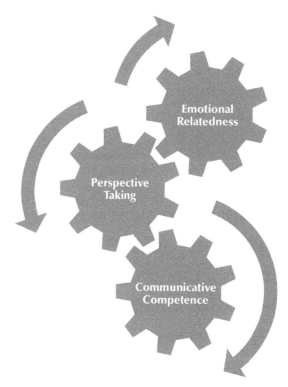

As children become young men and women, their emotional, social, economic, and physical well-being will be determined, in part, by their ability to grasp the Big Picture in social situations. As described above, there are many particulars involved, all of which are necessary aspects to include when creating an effective social curriculum. This book is written to help students to better understand social behaviors, perspective taking, communication, emotions, and the intricacies of relationships. Most important, it highlights the need to recognize that there are **many** parts that make up an experience and that each of these parts needs consideration when we are involved in and interpreting social experiences – a common area of challenge among individuals on the autism spectrum.

What Age Range Does the Book Target?

It is difficult to specify an age range for whom this book is most suitable. No two children with an autism spectrum diagnosis are exactly the same. This is so blaringly obvious that a higher-functioning student I once worked with wondered out loud, "Why do they call it Asperger Syndrome anyway? I mean, why do they lump us all together under the same name when we are all so different?" In many ways, he was correct.

Even with the increased interest in better serving students with ASD, many educators and professionals still frequently make the mistake of grouping all "autistic" youngsters together, without assessing what their needs truly are. Different students need different intervention strategies. Without the flexibility to use many different learning strategies, an intervention plan in any area, not just socialization, will most certainly be less effective. This happens often in a lot of educational settings, where resources are limited or prescribed by district administration personnel who have little clinical understanding of the population they are trying to service. This leaves teachers, or specialists, with nothing but the one "curriculum" that they are directed to use. Successful social-cognitive intervention strategies are generally a combination of many different types of goals, materials, and activities.

In order to ensure success, work with the ideas in this book requires guidance from an adult who knows the skill level of the student and how he or she learns. Most of the students I work with have considerable difficulty with carryover and generalization of the skills they learn. That is why I recommend either reading this book with the student or allowing the student to move through it independently, one chapter at a time, and then following up to determine how much, or how little, the student has learned and internalized.

Without the flexibility to use many different learning strategies, an intervention plan in any area, not just socialization, will most certainly be less effective.

This is especially important for children who tend to memorize information but fail to integrate what they know and demonstrate it in their everyday experiences. For example, many students with ASD can answer every social question correctly, yet they make mistakes in real life over and over again.

I work with a 13-year-old boy with high-functioning autism who has great academic skills. He is very bright, particularly in mathematics, and has a fantastic memory for factual information. This has helped him attain straight A's on his report card every year he has been in school. However, despite his abilities, he has a great deal of difficulty in the critical thinking areas, especially with inferential thinking, predicting, and applying the things he has learned in new situations. These weaknesses impact negatively his ability to take what he has learned about social skills and put those skills into practice.

We have the same conversations over and over about the mistakes that he continually makes when interacting with his peers. An area of great challenge for him is controlling his impulse to monitor the behaviors of other students in his class. He is the classic "rule police officer," letting everyone know, in various ways, what rules they are not following. When we get together for a session, he frequently relates stories about how this behavior has gotten him into "trouble" with teachers and students alike. When I ask him about what went wrong, he is always able to tell me the right answer. He recognizes, **after the fact**, that he was "too focused on the details" and not thinking flexibly, and that it's not his job "to be the rule police." Even so, he continues to have a great deal of difficulty integrating these things into a "social" situation.

While we struggle with "taking the show on the road," so to speak, I know from my observations that our work together has produced changes in his processing style, increased his abilities in the critical thinking areas, and improved his understanding of himself. What has made the most difference for him, aside from his work with me, is the involvement of his mother and other family members. They understand that working on social skills is a "24-hour-a day job" and that one group, once a week, is not enough. In order to support changes in the neurological profile of a child on the spectrum, practice is necessary. The students with the most familial involvement, those whose families understand their strengths and weaknesses, are the students who make the most progress.

Within my practice, I have successfully used this book with students between the ages of 6 and 24 years, with those who read and those who have limited reading abilities. After first assessing the student and making a determination about his or her abilities in each of the areas I intend to reinforce (ToM, emotional relatedness, and communicative competence, as well as abilities in holistic thinking), I determine if the presentation of the material within the book needs to be modified in some way. I have had to make adjustments for children who have difficulty with reading comprehension and language processing. These adjustments have included ...

- Adding more visual support to accompany the written material. This generally involves including more "pictures" or using photographs of the student and his or her personal experiences.

- Limiting the amount of information that is reviewed; for example, reading only one chapter at a time or even one or two skills within a chapter at a time.

- Adjusting the questions or providing verbal prompts to help the child to understand and answer the questions within the text.

- Reading the written material out loud to the student with appropriate pacing, emphasis, and emotion. Also, changing the "level" of the language and vocabulary (for example, substituting vocabulary words that are beyond the student's comprehension level) for better comprehension, either before reading or while reading.

While you might choose to use this book *with* the student, it is actually written for the students *themselves.* If you, as a parent or educator, decide to let a child read through the book on his own, a grade range of approximately fifth grade through high school is generally appropriate, depending on the student's developmental level and interest in the way the material is presented. Other things to consider include the student's reading comprehension level, overall language abilities, and ability to utilize critical thinking skills to respond to the examples and questions. If you are a parent and are unsure of whether your child can benefit from this book on a more independent level, consult a professional you trust and who knows your son or daughter, such as a teacher, a speech-language pathologist, or a psychologist.

How to Use This Book

Reading this book with the student or students you would like to support is an excellent way to help them internalize the material. Here are some things to remember when reading together:

- **Don't be a "teacher."** Think of this work as "shared" reading. Your job is to be the mediator between the student and the material. You won't be reading **to** them; you will be reading with them. You may be the only one reading if reading is difficult for the student you are working with, but you will need to stop along the way to discuss and check for comprehension.

- **Be familiar with the material ahead of time.** Read it to yourself first and be sure you fully understand the material. Think about how you will read it aloud to the student. Develop extension questions or comprehension questions as you prepare.

- **Use appropriate pacing, emphasis, and emotion.** Read the sections clearly and carefully to let the points sink in. Many words are in bold print, and these require more affect in order to highlight their importance for the student. Using appropriate affect while you read can help a student naturalistically obtain information about emotions.

- **Pay attention to the language.** Within the text, you might find vocabulary that you think may be difficult for the student you are working with. As these words come up, stopping to define or describe the words may be necessary. Keep track of the words and use them in context for the student to support thinking holistically. Also, highlight figurative language and words that have multiple meanings as they are used. These aspects of abstract language are generally difficult for our students. Again, focus on them as they appear in the context of the text and translate them into a context that is familiar to the student in order to encourage carryover.

- **Stop and ask questions.** Many questions are embedded within the chapters that you will be able to use, and you may create your own as you move along in order to check for comprehension. Use both open-ended and closed-set questions as you see fit. Give the student time to think about each question, but not so much that he forgets the point. Emphasize by pausing and making a "fresh start" when you are leaving one point and shifting topics. Otherwise, the student might mistake your words and think they are in response to his answers when, in fact, you are moving forward.

- **Think like the student.** The book is full of "thinking stories." Your presentation and attitude should reflect to the student that the important thing is to "think carefully" about the questions as opposed to knowing the answers immediately. For many questions, the answers will vary from student to student. And for many questions, there is more than one correct answer. See if students can think flexibly enough to come up with multiple responses on their own. If not, take the time to show them that there are possibilities they haven't considered.

- **Give positive reinforcement for thoughtful answers.** Many questions that you will be asking are "open-ended," meaning that there might not be *one* correct answer. Let students know what that means and explain that they won't get such answers wrong as long as they are thinking about it. Should students have a great deal of difficulty converging on an appropriate answer, point out to them, using visuals if necessary (this is where quick drawing skills come in), how they might "think about the question differently." Remind them that they are not "wrong" and praise them for doing a great job of following along and making an effort to come up with an answer.

Reading this book with the student or students you would like to support is an excellent way to help them internalize the material.

- **Think about thinking.** Ask students how they arrived at their answers to questions or what made them think about certain comments. Meta-cognitive skills (that is, thinking about thinking) are very important to the social skills process and to improvement in many learning areas. Students need to know how they arrived at an answer so that they can remember the process for the next time. Allow higher-functioning children to debate their answers with you or with each other. Working through challenging moments is important to the thinking process and also just good practice at handling differing opinions.

The way you interact with students when you read the material with them can make a big difference in how they attend, listen, retain, and recall the information.

If you choose to let your child, or a student you are working with, read this book independently, I urge you to still consider yourself a partner or mediator to the student throughout the process. Follow up with the student after he has read each chapter, or between concepts within a chapter. This will help to confirm the student's comprehension of the concepts and encourage generalization. **Repeated practice and reinforcement of the material is the best way to make changes in thought processes.**

Explain to students that they should think of this book as an ongoing project. Although it has a beginning, middle, and end, be sure to reinforce the idea that the dynamic nature of socialization frequently requires that you add to, subtract from, or, in other ways, alter the words and ideas presented. For example, you may find that the student you are working with becomes distracted or has difficulty with comprehension when reading some of the lengthier passages within a chapter.

In such a situation, it is helpful to focus on a visual and change the narrative into a bulleted list that includes the most salient information. Such simple adjustments can be done within a blank notebook or be prepared ahead of time on the computer. Also, adding relevant pictures or photographs with the student in them is also often helpful.

The activities at the end of each chapter allow students to practice the skills that have been introduced. Although some pages in and of themselves are "practice" worksheets, these activities are included as another way to support this type of social curriculum. These activities are appropriate for:

- One child to use independently and then review with adult support (parent or teacher)

- A teacher or other professional to use with a student on an individualized basis

- A professional to use within a social skills group

It is particularly important to review these practice ideas both before and after they are attempted and completed by the student(s) you are working with. Some things to remember:

- **Make sure that the student is clear about the directions for the activity.** Read the idea in the book and then clarify it with simpler language or visuals if needed.

- **Make sure that the student has all of the materials she needs, index cards, markers, pens, a notebook, journal, or whatever else is necessary to complete the activity.** This is especially important for students who have difficulty planning and organizing. You don't have to get everything for them, but you can prompt them to make a list of things they need before they get started.

- **Do some of the prep work ahead of time if you think it is necessary.** If the practice idea requires finding pictures of emotions on the Internet, you can make the activity easier by finding them yourself and providing choices to the student. If the student is able to, let her search and find pictures, which will make the activity a little more challenging.

- **If an activity says "with a partner," consider yourself the partner.** You can and should participate in the activity or game with the student, especially the first time around. Once the student understands the idea of a game, for example, you might try to facilitate him "playing" it with a peer. Participating in games with peers is generally more difficult for students than practicing with an adult. However, when they are working or playing with a peer, they are practicing the skill and also practicing "real-life" social interactions simultaneously and that is the true test of their skills.

The ideas presented in this book can and should be used in conjunction with other materials. As discussed above, no **one** curriculum, book, or methodology is appropriate for any **one** specific child. The works listed in the bibliography are useful to include in the intervention process.

Special Considerations for the Adults Using This Book

Although this book is written for children, it is also useful to adults who work or live with children who are diagnosed with autism or a similar disorder by providing information about what kind of skills to target and how to talk to students about them. In addition, practice exercises and suggestions for carryover activities are included, and these are critical ingredients for success.

I encourage parents and educators to use this book as a resource in the following ways:

- Use the book to help you gain a better understanding of what goals might be necessary to target and how to do so, for your child or the children you are working with.

- Use the book to help structure a social skills program. Use the activities at the end of each chapter as exercises within your program.

- Explain to the students you are working with what the book is about and how it can teach and help them remember what they need to know about social interactions. This will support their self-awareness, as well as be a good learning tool for them to refer to when needed.

- Read the book with the child and talk about the topics on each page. Use examples from the child's own real-life experiences to help her further understand the application of the material. Also, use examples from your own experiences to show how you solved similar problems.

- Make the book available for future "planning" moments. For example, use it to review skills and situations ahead of time, such as before a play-date for a young child or before a school dance for a teenager. Hopefully, this will make their social attempts more successful.

- Use the book when the child has faced challenging moments with friends, in school, or other activities, to review what he or she might have done differently.

- Make new pages for the book to personalize it. Add topics that are specific to a given child's needs. Use the format of this guide to help you write the additional information.

Using visual supports with the students in my groups has been a very effective way of helping them retain and internalize the information presented. In addition, students often become so connected to the visuals that they themselves begin to draw or write as a tool to communicate about experiences that they have had. This can further engage them in conversation and the learning experience as a whole. The written word, pictures, drawings, and meaningful colors further reinforce verbal information and often serve as a record to refer back to and to provide further opportunities to connect.

If you are a parent or professional working with a person or a child with social challenges and you are using this book, I highly recommend keeping a blank notebook or sketchpad and a set of markers of various colors close at hand. This way, as you discuss situations or work through the book, you can personalize the material, using information about the students themselves. Drawing pictures is very helpful for those who have more significant problems with auditory comprehension of language. You don't need to be artistic; stick figures work just fine. For more details about how to make this work, use the words and pictures in this book as a model or refer to Carol Gray's excellent resources, *The New Social Stories™ Book: 10th Anniversary Edition* (2010) or *Comic Strip Conversations* (1994).

How the Book Is Organized

The organization of this book reflects a developmental approach, and the order of certain topics is not arbitrary. For example, developmental information tells us that babies begin to pick up on non-verbal communication as early as 5 months of age. So, information about these important precursors to verbal communication appears within this book prior to the information about verbal communication skills.

However, social learning is a parallel, not a sequential, process. That is why the skills and ideas in this area overlap and need to be continually reinforced to encourage generalization. Social learning is ongoing. Creating and recognizing teaching moments should be an active part of life for the adults who support children with social skills deficits, and these should reflect the ever-changing nature of social interactions. This too supports the child's understanding and integration of the social environment as they get older.

> Creating and recognizing teaching moments should be an active part of life for the adults who support children with social skills deficits, and these should reflect the ever-changing nature of social interactions.

The Big Picture

Arriving at the Big Picture is not as easy as adding up each skill and then automatically knowing what to do. For a child with social deficits, it can be a painstaking task. While it may be harder for some and easier for others, it is effortful for all. The level of impairment in other areas further complicates weaknesses in central coherence, including theory of mind, motivation, emotional regulation, language skills, sensory difficulties, and self-regulation. All of these factors contribute to the relative success of the child.

This book alone does not provide all the answers to the questions we have about the children we work with. But the information and examples presented here can serve as an essential "road map" to finding social success. Most important, it will enhance a child's self-understanding, which is an invaluable tool for success all future endeavors.

Why Should I Read This Book? An Introduction for Students

How Did I Get Here?

Right now, you are probably reading this book with an adult you know and trust. This could be a teacher, therapist, parent, or friend. Or, you are reading this book by yourself in order to get ready to talk about it with an adult. Maybe you have been to a "social skills group," where discussions and activities about social skills are planned and carried out.

Take a minute and think about how you got started reading this book. Yes, that's right. Take a minute and think …

Learning Happens Everywhere

Some people think that learning happens only in school or in "school-like" places, like church or synagogue, music lessons, or sports training. Most people think, "If I am being taught by someone else, then I must be learning something."

It's true that you can learn a lot that way, but there are times when **you are your own** teacher, such as when you get a new video game and you "teach" yourself how to play it. That is a "learn as you go" kind of learning. Video games are easy to learn by yourself. You try out a new route to the castle to save the princess, and run into a dragon that eats you and takes one of your lives. No big deal, you can try another path with another one of your lives. Learning to drive a car, on the other hand, is harder, and it requires a teacher.

Sometimes you think you can teach yourself, but then you realize that what you are working on is too hard and you need some help after all. You might think that you can teach yourself how to drive; however, once you get into the car and drive it into the pond next to your house, you'll know you have to find someone to help you. Remember, in real life, you don't have an unlimited number of lives like in a video game.

Learning social skills is something that you might think is no big deal to handle by yourself, but it can be a big deal. And, if you're like a lot of other people who need help with social skills, you might not know how to ask for that help, or even be able to see that you do need help. **You are reading this book because someone who is close to you thinks it is important that you read it.**

What Are Social Skills Anyway and How Do We Learn Them?

Social skills are learned behaviors that allow you to interact and communicate with other people. "**Social learning**" is watching, learning, and remembering what to do in social situations. You can probably think of some "social rules" that were taught to you, maybe by your parents saying things such as, "Don't pick on your little sister so much!" or "Take turns with those toys or I'm taking them away!" Or maybe your teacher reminded you about the "rules" in the classroom. For example, "Raise your hand if you want to talk." "Use an inside voice in the classroom." or "Don't yell out the answers."

Most of how we communicate and interact with other people is picked up more "automatically" as we make connections and form relationships with others. For example, you probably learned about what kinds of things your best friend likes to do just from hanging out together over a period of time – not because he gave you a list to memorize on the day you met. You learned about him by observing, thinking, remembering, and simply being with him. This is how much social learning takes place.

Everyone Is Different

Maybe it's not easy for you to observe and remember the things that your friend likes to do, as in the example above. Maybe you need to be reminded about how to stay focused on your friend when you are with him, so that you don't ignore his interests and only talk about what you like. Imagine getting together with a friend who loves playing a video game that you hate, and he won't stop talking about it or playing it when you are with him. How do you think that will make you feel? Bored? Annoyed? Frustrated? Angry? Maybe you feel all of those …

Even though we said that most social learning is picked up automatically, that is not always the case. Some people may know just the right thing to say to a friend, and others may be good at communicating feelings with their faces. However, if you are reading this book, it's likely that you are having some difficulty with social learning. Or, maybe you have learned certain social skills but are having trouble "performing" them when you need to. Reading this book is one way of helping you learn how to be more successful socially.

Be the Change You Want to See

This book is like a handbook for thinking about being "social:" that is, interacting with others in many different ways. It describes important things to pay attention to when you are with others so they want to be around you and so your work or play goes more smoothly, like remembering what your friends are interested in, understanding emotions, and sharing and working cooperatively with others. These are the rules that most people learn automatically.

It also includes some "unwritten rules" that are important to remember in particular situations, like the fact that most kids in middle school don't think it's cool to wear Spongebob Squarepants t-shirts because they think it's childish. Thinking about these rules can be helpful. But don't worry about remembering everything in this book. You can always come back to it in the future.

Getting the Main Idea: Big Picture Thinking

There's nothing wrong with having a hard time learning something or needing extra help. Everyone has things they are good at and things that are hard for them. If learning social skills is something that is hard for you, I'm here to give you one **BIG** clue about what to do. I have had a lot of experience working with people who have a difficult time with social skills. I have learned a lot of different "tips and tricks" that I want you to know about, and that's why I wrote this book.

Lots of times people have a hard time with socializing because they are paying too much attention to the "little things" that are happening around them, and not enough attention to how those little things fit into something bigger. Focusing too much on details can cause you to forget that those details are part of a larger whole. Think of a jigsaw puzzle ... if you only look at the individual pieces you cannot see the finished product – the Big Picture – they are supposed to fit into.

This book is written to help you remember to think about all the details in a situation and then see how those details fit into your whole social experience. Remembering to focus on the "whole," and not just the little things, is sometimes called "getting the Big Picture."

Not everyone is a Big Picture Thinker, but when it comes to social skills, being a Big Picture Thinker can really help you out.

Big Picture Thinkers are people who:

- **Think flexibly and know that there can be more than one way to solve a problem.**

- **Understand that there doesn't always have to be a "correct" or right way to do something.**

- **Learn from every experience they have – both successes and failures – and use the information that they have learned to help them with future challenges.**

- **Know that they need to try a lot of different things, take some chances, and then take the time to learn from both their positive and negative experiences.**

- **Learn from the others around them about how they can contribute to the group.**

The main goal of this book is to get you thinking about social skills and to help you be a better observer of yourself and the people you are interacting with. It will also give you ideas about how to practice what you are learning. Being more aware of how what you are learning fits into real life is an important goal. It's not just about knowing "what to do:" it's "how you do it" that really counts. This book will help you put your knowledge and your actions together into a more manageable "whole." It's called the **Big Picture** for just that reason.

This book may also do a lot of other important things for you. I hope that it will:

- Help you better understand your strengths and weaknesses, and how to use your strengths to help you.

- Help you organize your thoughts and feelings about relationships and assist you in being more successful when interacting with others.

- Help you better understand your own emotions and learn the importance of understanding the emotions of others.

- Become an important reference book for your future use.

Finally, I hope this book will help you to make changes in your social interactions. Before you begin, take a minute to make a picture in your head of something that you would really like to accomplish. Visualize yourself doing exactly what you want to do … **BE the change you wish to see**. This book can help!

Getting Started With Big Picture Thinking

This book describes important things that you need to think about when trying to improve your social behavior. Each chapter outlines a concept such as emotions or self-control. Those bigger concepts consist of smaller parts that I call *place, person, face-to-face,* and *word clues* that will be introduced in Chapter 1.

The chapters move along in this way:

1. First, the "whole idea" is introduced (like emotions or self-control) along with many of the pieces that make up that whole. This should help you get a picture in your mind about what will be discussed within the chapter.

2. Next, a story example called Kids in Action is presented to help you see how the pieces that will be discussed fit together within the chapter concept.

3. At the end of each chapter, you will find a review, along with some ideas for how you can practice what you have learned. **Practice is important when learning new skills of any kind, and this is no different for social skills.**

4. You will also see a picture that looks like this at the end of each chapter:

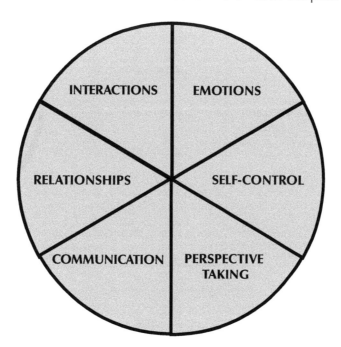

The circle above represents how social interactions consist of many different parts that make up a whole situation and shows that it is important to think about all of them. As you read through each chapter, at the end of the chapter, you will see another piece of the circle revealed. This will help to remind you of the importance of Big Picture Thinking.

If you can understand the concept parts as they are discussed and think about how they fit together in a whole situation, then you will be seeing the Big Picture. Once you have a better grasp of what the whole situation is about, you can be more socially successful.

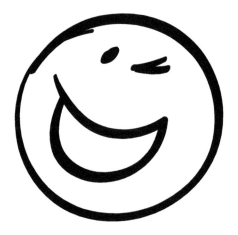

Important Note: Each chapter is only a "guide." Social situations are **NOT** the same every time. You can start with what is written here, and then see how the pieces fit within your own experiences.

It would be impossible to write a book about every kind of social experience that you will have. It is difficult to plan ahead for something that **might** happen. Not only that, this book may describe a certain kind of experience, or provide an example or story that is similar to your own experiences: however, there is no real way for it to be exactly like your life. It is for these reasons that you are probably working with an adult as you read this book. An adult can help you connect the information in the book to your own life, until you can start recognizing the similarities and differences yourself.

Kids in Action

Below is the first Kids in Action story. You will see one at the beginning of every chapter, right after the topic of the chapter has been introduced. The story relates to the skills in the chapter, and it describes a real social situation. Sometimes the characters get it right, and sometimes they don't. The questions that follow will get you thinking further about the story, the skills involved, and the Big Picture. And guess what … if you can get the main idea of the stories, you will be able to say that you are getting better at being a Big Picture Thinker.

 KIDS IN ACTION: AN INTRODUCTION TO THE BIG PICTURE

Marisa and Hayley are best friends. They spend a lot of time together at school and at each other's homes. At school, they enjoy making up their own games at recess time. Sometimes Marisa is the one to create the game, and sometimes Hayley is. They know each other well, so no matter who makes the suggestion, they can easily get started playing.

Today during lunch, Hayley suggested that they pretend to be movie stars filming a movie. Marisa thought it was a good idea and suggested using the playhouse at the top of the climbing structure as a "dressing room." Both girls were able to quickly see how the story might develop and how they might add to it, without talking too much about the details. When they got to the playground, their story took off and went on until the whistle was blown to come inside.

The next day, another friend, Jackie, sat with Marisa and Hayley at lunchtime. The girls suggested that she join their "Movie Star" game during recess. Both Marisa and Hayley like Jackie, but sometimes it's not so easy to get started playing with her. Jackie liked the idea of the game and agreed to play with them. Once the three got out to the playground, Jackie began to ask a lot of questions about what was going to happen. She was very focused on the details of what was happening within the story, like what their "movie star names" were going to be, where they were filming, what time of the day it was, who was going to be the director … and so on. Jackie did not seem to be able to get started until all the details were figured out the way that she thought they should be. Hayley, Marisa, and Jackie spent so much time talking that before they even got started playing, the whistle was blown, and recess was over.

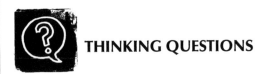

THINKING QUESTIONS

Why did it take the girls so long to get started playing their game after Jackie joined them?

Which of these three girls seems to have the most difficulty seeing the Big Picture?

How do you think Hayley and Marisa felt about including Jackie to their game?

Do you think Marisa and Hayley are likely to include Jackie in their next game?

REWIND

You may have noticed a difference between how Marisa, Hayley, and Jackie were able to "get into the game." Marisa and Hayley were able to see the whole idea of the pretend play, but Jackie had a more difficult time with it. She seemed to get stuck on the little details before she even started playing, whereas Marissa and Hayley were able to let those details happen naturally while they were playing.

In this example, Jackie's difficulty with Big Picture Thinking has affected the girls' interactions negatively. They can't get started playing in time to enjoy their game and each other.

Chapter 1

The Big Picture: What Is It?

The Big Picture is a way to describe how important it is to think about your social interactions as a "whole."

There are many things you need to understand about yourself and the part you play when interacting with others. Many small details make up the Big Picture in a social situation.

Here are some of the things you need to think about (see also pages A2-A3):

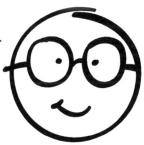

Place Clues -This means you are thinking about the physical environment around you.
- Where are you?
- What's going on around you?
- What kind of behavior is appropriate for the place you are in?

People Clues – This means you are thinking about the people that are around you.
- What is your relationship to the people you are with?
- What is your understanding of your own mood or feelings?
- What is your understanding of the feelings and point of view of the others around you?

Face-to-Face Clues – This means thinking about the nonverbal cues displayed by others.
- What are the people around you saying with their body language, gestures, facial expressions, and eye gaze? Do these visual cues match what they are saying?
- What is their appearance like? Clothes, hair, skin color, height, and weight are all important.
- What does their voice sound like?

Word Clues – This means thinking about what is being said.
- What are the other people around you saying?
- Do their words match what you think they might be feeling?

KIDS IN ACTION: THE BIG PICTURE, WHAT IS IT?

Avery is late getting to science class. Since he arrived late, he doesn't know that the teacher has given an assignment that needs to be done in small work groups. When he approaches the doorway, he can see that the students have moved their desks together so that they can complete their work and no one is talking above a whisper.

Usually when Avery walks into science, he calls out a "hello" to his teacher and friends, walks to his desk, and "chats" with the person who sits next to him in his regular speaking voice until the bell rings and the teacher starts a whole class discussion. Today, something clearly different is going on, and if Avery chooses to enter the room in the usual way, he might disrupt the class.

 THINKING QUESTIONS

This is a good time for Avery, or anyone, to consider the situation he is in as a whole. If he focuses on the "usual" details, he will miss what's really happening. The details are things like:

- What are the people around Avery doing?

- What are their faces or bodies saying?

- Where is the teacher and what is she focused on?

- Does Avery hear the people around him talking? What are they saying?

 REWIND

Once Avery has a good idea about everything that is happening around him, he can make a choice about how to deal with this new experience without disrupting others.

Chapter 1 Review: The Big Picture: What Is It?

This chapter introduced the concept of the Big Picture and described what this book is about. Now that you know what to expect, you are better prepared to learn and practice. I hope you can already see how the information in the book will be helpful to you in social interactions.

It may be a good idea to have a blank notebook next to you while you read, so you can write down any questions, comments, or thoughts that you have. You can also use the notebook for doing some of the practice exercises that are listed at the end of each chapter. Keeping everything together in one place is important: Stay organized so you can go back and look at it again when you need or want to.

In this chapter, you learned more about Big Picture Thinking. You read the example of Avery and how he needed to put all the clues (or details) – person, place, face-to-face, and word clues – together before he made a decision about what to do when entering the classroom. The practice exercises below will help you further with big picture thinking.

 # Practice Ideas

Students: On the next page are some activities you can do that will help you practice thinking about the Big Picture as it has been introduced in this chapter. It probably looks like a lot of work, but don't worry, you don't have to do all of them at once. Pick one to start with and then review it with an adult who is helping you both before and after you have completed it. You can always come back to the practice activities again later to do more. Don't forget, practice makes perfect.

Parents and Educators: In the introduction, you read some suggestions regarding supporting a student through the practice activities. It might be helpful to review them again after you read the paragraph below.

Consider the practice activities at the end of each chapter "extension" activities that will help reinforce the material in each chapter. If you have chosen to let a student read the material independently, it is a good idea to review the material she has read before getting started on the activities. Review the practice activity with the student to make sure she understands what it entails and then allow her to complete it. If it is a role-play, you will be able to participate. If it is a written activity, try letting the student finish it independently and then review it together. Ask the student to explain what she wrote and why. Letting the student verbalize what she has done will help reinforce a more holistic thinking style, and it will also help encourage carryover.

If the student you are working with needs more support, go through each practice activity with her, eliciting responses as a "mediator," not a teacher. If handwriting is an issue for the student, ask her to verbalize the responses while you serve as a scribe or have her use a computer instead of a notebook.

1. **Create a "timeline" of your life.** Start at the beginning and include events that are significant for you. Include predictions for "future" important events, even though they haven't actually happened. Be sure to share your timeline with someone and explain.

2. **Develop a classified ad.** Pretend you need to advertise yourself and your personality so that others will have a better idea of who you are. Write a newspaper classified ad describing yourself. In only three lines, tell the reader about you. This can be the Big Picture about you.

3. **Explain and describe.** Find someone to talk with, like an adult or a friend, and briefly explain the **main idea** of this book, the Big Picture, as if you were recommending it to somebody. Think about the person you are talking with, have they read the book? If not, you need to give enough detail so they understand what you mean, but not too many details so that they don't lose interest in what you are saying.

4. **See the "main idea."** Practice talking about the "main idea" by describing your favorite activity, TV show, movie, etc., to someone. Use the guidelines in #3 above to help you remember how.

   Here are some other things you can explain or describe using Big Picture Thinking:
   - Explain to your teacher why you did not do your homework last night. Create an excuse that you think the teacher has never heard before.
   - Describe a holiday that no one has ever heard of before.
   - Explain the wrong way to prepare for a really important test.
   - Describe a "magic potion" that you have created and talk about the special powers it has.
   - Describe the worst gift that you have ever received and what you did with it.
   - Describe what you would do to your bedroom if you had a chance to change it completely and money was no object.

Chapter 2

The Big Picture: Feelings and Emotions

I n this chapter, you will be thinking about feelings and emotions. Understanding feelings and emotions is an important part of being able to see the Big Picture. You need to be able to:

- Label the feelings you have using emotion words

- Understand that there are many different emotions

- Understand that everyone's emotional experiences are different

- Recognize that there are "levels" of feelings

- Express your feelings appropriately to others

- Appropriately deal with the emotions you experience

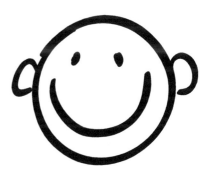

Also, you need to think about the feelings and emotions of other people. This is important because you need to be able to:

- Recognize what people around you are feeling and experiencing

- Label others' feelings with emotion words

- Understand the "level" of the feeling that someone is expressing

- Deal with the emotions of others around you

- Recognize that your behavior has an effect on other people and pay attention to this so you can change your behavior if necessary

KIDS IN ACTION: FEELINGS AND EMOTIONS

Brooke and Tessa are sisters. Brooke is 12 and Tessa is 10. Their family does a lot of things together, and they especially enjoy taking a family vacation every summer. Brooke has been asking her parents to plan a trip to Disney World, but every time she makes the suggestion, Tessa gets extremely upset and starts to cry. She says she has no interest in going to Disney World, and usually they end up having a big argument. Sometimes she yells at Brooke and says things like, "You don't understand my feelings at all!" Brooke sees that Tessa is upset, but she has no idea why visiting Disney World would cause a tantrum. Brooke responds, "How can I understand your feelings at all if you won't talk about them? What about my feelings? I want to go to Disney and all of your complaining isn't helping."

Finally, Brooke and her parents become completely frustrated, and they push Tessa to explain. She says she's afraid of the dressed-up "characters" that walk around the park. She is worried that if they went to Disney World, she might see, or have to be close to, one of them, and that would really upset her. Brooke can't understand why Tessa can't just ignore the characters and enjoy the rest of the attractions and rides, but Tessa is sure that she will be too afraid to think about anything else.

Tessa's parents tell her how proud they are that she shared these difficult feelings with them. Then they tell her how much they care about her and how they want to help her deal with these difficult feelings so that the whole family can have a really fantastic and exciting vacation together.

Getting support from her parents makes Tessa want to try to figure out a solution to her problem. They have shown her that her feelings are important and that they will help her try to make the changes she needs to make so that the whole family can be happy. Tessa now realizes that the feelings of her family members are important too, and that makes her want to change even more.

 THINKING QUESTIONS

What was Tessa's problem? What was Brooke's problem?

Why didn't Tessa tell her sister or her parents what she was feeling right from the beginning?

How do you think Tessa's parents felt about this situation?

Have you ever had an experience where it was difficult to tell someone about what you were feeling?

 REWIND

In this story, Tessa was dealing with feelings of fear and worry that were very overwhelming to her. She had difficulty labeling her feelings, expressing them to others appropriately, and managing her behavior in response to them. Her feelings were so "big" that she refused to go on a family vacation to Disney World, something that should have been fun and easy for her.

In this chapter, we will review emotion words. Specifically, we will talk about how to recognize feelings and start to talk about examples of what types of situations might make you feel a certain way.

Understanding Feelings and Emotions

Emotions are a combination of physical feelings and mental thoughts. They are the feelings that you have during a situation or experience. They are a personal experience … different for everyone. Emotions and feelings go together as your body and mind experience things.

A feeling can also be a description of a physical reaction to what is happening around you, or inside of you. The senses in all parts of your body receive information that is sent to your brain, where you think about what's happening now and compare it to other experiences that you have had in the past. Then your mind and body react in an emotional and physical way. You might have a "feeling of warmth" inside when someone acts kindly toward you, or you might feel "sick inside" when you are dealing with a situation that is making you nervous, like taking a test or performing in a play.

No one has the same reactions, or feelings, in response to a situation. How you feel has a lot to do with how you usually react to something, or how the situation relates to your past experiences.

For example, maybe you had a bad experience the first time you rode on a rollercoaster at an amusement park. Since that time, you have not been able to ride a rollercoaster because you are too frightened or nervous about the height or the speed.

Now, suppose you go on a trip to an amusement park with friends and they suggest going on the newest, fastest, tallest roller coaster in the park. Chances are your memories will affect your current emotional state, making you too **nervous** to ride at all, or possibly feeling **horrified** afterward if you do choose to ride. Your friends may feel completely different. They may feel **excited** about riding or completely **energized** afterward. In the Kids in Action story at the beginning of this chapter, Tessa's fear of "characters" made her nervous about a possible trip to Disney, while her sister Brooke felt very excited about that kind of a vacation.

It is important to pay attention to how your body feels in different situations. You will pick up a lot of important clues that way that will help you better understand the Big Picture of what is happening around you. For example, you may notice that your body or face gets hot very quickly when the teacher calls on you in class and you don't know an answer. This feeling in your body might have to do with the fact that you are **worried** about being singled out in front of your friends or **nervous** about your performance in class. Or you might feel your cheeks become warm when you are blushing because of feeling **embarrassed**.

Paying attention to your emotions will help you understand what you are feeling and communicate that to others when it is necessary.

When you understand your emotions and yourself, and know how to express yourself in response to your feelings, you can make better decisions about your social interactions.

Feeling Thermometer

A **Feeling Thermometer** is a tool you can use to help you understand your feelings. It gives you a way to "see" how much of a certain feeling you are experiencing and help you create a clearer picture in your mind about your feelings.

A real thermometer measures your body's temperature. When your body temperature goes up, you can see it on the thermometer. In the same way, a Feeling Thermometer measures how you are experiencing a particular feeling in a situation.

The Feeling Thermometer can help you "measure" how "big" or "small" your feelings are in different situations. Then, you can think about how you might deal with future experiences that make you feel the same way. You can draw a picture of a thermometer or use the one in the Appendix on page A4 of this book, and draw in the "mercury" (the red line) where you think it should be to show the level of your feelings.

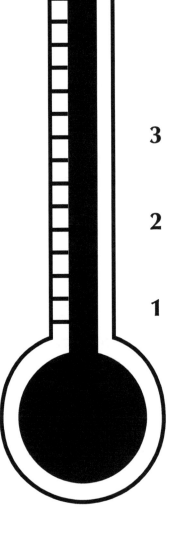

For example, suppose you are thinking about being frustrated and what situations make you feel frustrated. You could use the thermometer picture to represent a situation like "rules that mom and dad make that I don't agree with" and then draw in the "red" to show how much frustration, or how little, you feel.

Seeing "how much" frustration you are feeling can make it easier for you to think about and talk about your feelings. You will also be more prepared as these situations come up again in the future. Then you will be able to choose a positive way to deal with the frustration you are feeling, like using a calming strategy or communicating and negotiating with your mom or dad, instead of having an argument.

When mom or dad makes a rule I don't agree with, my anger is at a 10.

The Incredible 5-Point Scale

The Incredible 5-Point Scale (Buron & Curtis, 2003) is another great tool that is similar to the Feeling Thermometer. It can help you "check in" on how you are feeling or what your behavior is in response to a feeling, or within a situation.

Suppose you want to take a closer look at how nervous or anxious you are when you are meeting someone new. On the scale, you would assign each number to a level of anxiety or nervousness. Number 1 describes how you are when you are not feeling nervous, and number 5 would be the most nervous and out of control.

For this example, the chart might read something like this:

    5   =   Out-of-control nervous, not able to meet new people.

    4   =   Really nervous, hands shaking, palms sweaty, need to try a calming strategy.

    3   =   Nervous, but not having any physical reactions.

    2   =   Nervous about possibly feeling nervous.

    1   =   Completely in control of feelings. Calm

You can also add pictures to help give you clues about how you are feeling, as illustrated below.

After the chart is complete, keep it around to refer back to and "check in" about how you are feeling before, during, or after you are in the situation you have described. There is a blank scale on page A5 of the Appendix you can fill in yourself.

From *The Incredible 5-Point Scale* by Kari Dunn Buron and Mitzi Curtis, 2003, Shawnee Mission, KS: AAPC Publishing. Reprinted with permission.

Emotions Vocabulary

Emotions can be labeled with words that help you, and other people, understand what you are feeling.

Keeping a list of words that describe and identify different emotions is helpful when you are trying to identify and talk about what you are feeling.

For some feelings, there are more than one word to describe them. These words allow you to describe different feelings within the same **"emotion family."** For example, "sad" can also be described as "unhappy," "upset," or "depressed."

The words in an emotion family are good tools to describe how much of a feeling you are experiencing and for how long. You can put the words in order, just like you did with the numbers on the Feeling Thermometer and the Incredible 5-Point Scale. For example, "depressed" is a label for a feeling that is "bigger" than sad. You might use it to describe how you are feeling when you are really unhappy for a long time. "Surprised" is an emotion that usually describes a reaction to something that is unexpected. It can be positive or negative, and it usually lasts for a short period of time. When a feeling of surprise continues for a longer period of time, it may be labeled and considered "shock," which would describe a feeling that is "bigger" than "surprised," lasting for a long period of time.

The next pages in this chapter will give you more information about emotion words. Sometimes the word "emotions" is used, and sometimes the word "feelings" is used. Regardless of which word is used, know that you should be thinking about your emotional experiences as a whole.

Each section defines an emotion. It will give you some details about what that emotion might feel or look like, describe some situations that might bring about that emotion, and list some synonyms (words that mean the same thing) and antonyms (opposites) related to the emotion word, that you might want to add to your vocabulary.

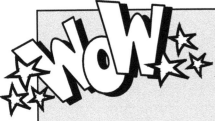

Remember: Not every single emotion is listed here, nor is every single word for each emotion ... to do that would take forever. It will be your job to start with what's here and then move forward with your own "emotion studies." For example, you can go through a dictionary and make a list of new emotion words.

Affection

Affection describes a feeling of fondness or love for a person you are close to, or a favorite pet. It usually describes a feeling that you have that is more than just friendship.

Affection is a connection that you have with other people that makes you feel good inside. Physically, you might feel warmth in your face or body when you are around another person for whom you feel affection. The physical reaction (feeling warmth) is a sign that you are feeling affection.

Understanding your relationship with someone will help you understand whether your feelings toward them are "more than friendly." You probably have feelings of great affection for your **parents, siblings, and other family members.** These are very close relationships where people express their connection to each other in a physical way, like hugging and kissing. You probably know for sure that your family members feel the same way about you because they have told you, and they probably have expressed their affection physically.

A best friend, or a boyfriend or girlfriend might also be people that you feel affection toward. Best friends also give you clues about their feelings through their words and possibly hugs (or other types of appropriate touching like putting their arm around you when they want to come in close to tell you a secret) for support or encouragement.

Talking with another person about how you feel about them will help you understand if they feel the same way. Looking for clues from their body language or facial expressions, such as how close they are sitting to you or where they are looking, when they are near you is another way to identify whether they feel affection toward you. That is, feeling affectionate can make you want to share with others by getting closer to them physically. You might want to talk about the connection you are experiencing, or you might want to hug, kiss, or touch the person or pet that you are feeling loving toward.

Wanting to be physically closer to the "object of your affection" is a typical feeling for most people.

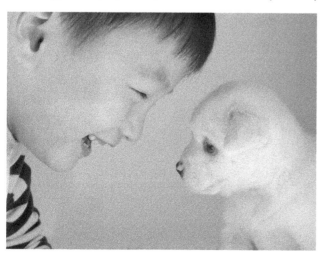

But it is important to make sure that you share your feelings of affection appropriately. This means you should be sure that the person you want to get close to is also feeling that kind of closeness for you on a regular basis. You also need to be sure that they are feeling ready to receive a hug (or kiss or touch) at the time that you are feeling ready to give it. In Chapter 6, we talk about levels of relationships. **Our closest relationships are the ones that are most appropriate for showing physical affection.**

It is usually appropriate to show and share affectionate feelings with family members, but not always in public. For example, you might feel comfortable giving a younger sibling a hug when you are at home, but not so comfortable doing it when you are in front of your friends. The same can be said for a parent. You might give your mom or dad a kiss at home, but not when they are dropping you off at school.

Your age has a lot to do with how you feel about expressing affection toward the people you are fond of. Younger children generally want to be physically closer to their parents and other family members, and they kiss, hug, sit on a lap, or hold hands for much of the time they are with the person they are connected to. As you grow, these things become less frequent.

Also, in our culture, girls usually express feelings of affection in a physical way more than boys. They tend to hug their best girlfriends more, walk hand in hand, or keep their arms around each other much more than boys do with each other.

This is usually true for most girls no matter what age they are. Around the second grade, boys stop hugging other boys that they are close with and tend to express feelings of affection toward their best friends through pats on the back or high fives.

Here are some sentences with words that describe "levels" or "degrees" of affection:

Warmth: Describing strong affection and kindness: "There was warmth in his greeting and handshake."

Fondness: Suggests a liking for something or someone: "She has a fondness for sweets so she always has candy in her desk drawer."

Love: Suggests a very strong feeling of warm personal attachment or deep affection: "I'm so proud of my niece Sammi, and I love her with all my heart!"

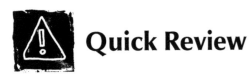 # Quick Review

What Is Affection?

- A happy feeling of fondness or love for a person or favorite pet
- Usually describes a relationship that is more than just friendship

How Does Affection Feel?

- That you are connected with other people, and that makes you feel good inside

- Warmth in your face or body when you are around another person can signal you feel affectionate toward him or her. The physical reaction (feeling warmth) is a sign that you are feeling affection.

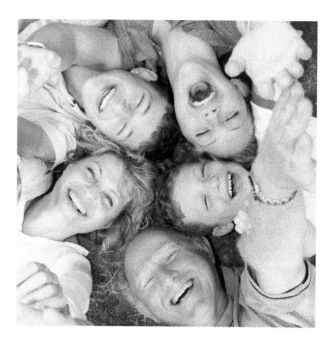

Body Language and Facial Expression Clues

Affection looks a lot like happiness:

- Smiling, with a closed or open mouth, with or without teeth showing.

- Big smiles make the cheeks look "round" or puffy.

- Muscles near the eyes squeeze the eyelids tighter.

- Smile muscles and eye muscles move with the same amount of intensity. IF NOT, the smile may be a fake smile.

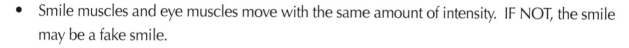

Affection Vocabulary

Synonyms (similar to) – fondness, tenderness, attachment, attraction, admiration, sensitivity, connectedness, warmth, love, appreciation, favor, adoration, devotion.

Antonyms (opposite of) – cold, distant, unfeeling, disapproval, disgust, dislike, hatred, aversion, contempt, loathing.

Anger

Anger is an unpleasant experience, where you disagree with someone or something. Anger may or may not be expressed outwardly. In other words, when you're angry you are probably not feeling great about the people or things around you. You might express these feelings to others or you might not.

You express anger, through your facial expressions, body language (which includes physically aggressive behavior), the words you speak, and physical changes in your body. Anger is a feeling that **everyone** experiences; however, not everyone deals with, or expresses, anger in the same way.

Anger can be healthy, because it may motivate you to make changes in your own behavior that will keep you safe physically and emotionally. For example, suppose you sit with the same kids every day at lunch. They think it's funny to throw pieces of food at a boy they think is kind of weird. You don't think it's funny at all. In fact, their behavior makes you mad. Since it doesn't feel great being angry every day at lunch, your feelings may get you to do something, like changing your seat or telling your friends how lousy you think they are for what they are doing. In this situation, your anger might be doing you a favor.

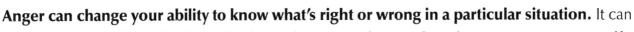

Anger can be an intense (very strong) feeling. When you are angry, your body usually goes through some physical changes. Your heartbeat and breathing get quicker, your face gets red or hot, and your muscles might become tense. How your body reacts depends on how angry you are as well as other experiences you have had. **Not everyone feels the same way when they are angry.**

Anger can change your ability to know what's right or wrong in a particular situation. It can happen very quickly, and this can lead to making poor choices about how you express yourself.

Going back to the lunch example, suppose you get angry with your friends for throwing food, and instead of making a calm decision to change seats, you react differently. Maybe you take your bottle of water and throw it at the guys you are sitting with. Maybe that bottle is full, and it soaks not just the guys, but also the teacher who is standing behind them. In this case, your response to your anger has caused an even bigger problem. So, again, it is important to first recognize that you are angry and then decide on an effective way of expressing it. In this case, moving away from the friends at lunch is an effective way of dealing with the issue: throwing a water bottle and hitting a teacher is not!

It's definitely okay to be angry. It's how you choose to express your anger that will affect you and the people around you the most. That is why it's important to know when you are feeling angry and then try to take some time to make a useful choice about what to do.

Steps You Can Take to Help You When You Are Angry

- Think about how your body is feeling and identify that you are angry – use the Feeling Thermometer or the 5-Point Scale, for example.

- Try to determine how angry you are.

- Try to stay calm and in control. If you need to, ask a grownup or a friend you really trust for help.

- Get away from what is making you angry, at least for a little while.

- Express your feelings – to a grownup or the person who is making you angry.

- Use an "I feel" statement when you want to express how you feel to someone. If you want to let them know that what they are doing is making you feel angry, you can say something like, "When you do ____, it really makes me feel angry. I would like you to stop." Using the lunch example again, you might say something like, "When you guys throw food at other people, it really makes me mad. Please stop doing it, or I won't be able to eat with you any more."

Examples of sentences that describe feelings of anger include: "He was yelling so loud that I knew he was feeling very angry about the situation," and "Although she was feeling angry about the decision, she kept it inside."

Here are some sentences with words that describe "levels" or "degrees" of anger:

Rage: Loss of self-control due to very angry feelings: "He was screaming with **rage**."

Fury: Destructive rage that might be seen by others as out of control: "In their **fury**, they smashed all the dishes."

Wrath: Desire to gain revenge or to punish another person: "In his **wrath**, the king ordered all the peasants to the dungeon."

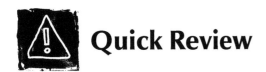

Quick Review

What Is Anger?

- An unpleasant feeling of being against someone or something

- An emotion that is sometimes expressed outwardly through words, facial expressions and/or body language

How Does Anger Feel?

- Rapid heartbeat

- Rapid breathing

- Paleness or redness (flushing) and warmth in the face.

- Tense muscles throughout the body

- Clenched fists

Body Language and Facial Expression Clues for Anger

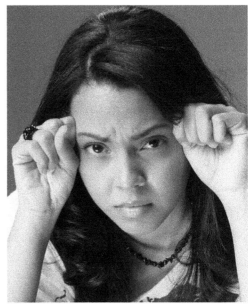

- Eyebrows lower and eyes open wider as anger gets "bigger"

- Glaring – eyelids pulled back almost touching the lower part of the eyebrows, a frown or a scowl on the face

- Paleness or flushed cheeks

- Change in voice volume

- Tense body postures – clenched fists or other tension in the body

- Facial expressions may change quickly when someone is angry, especially when they are also communicating verbally

---

Anger Vocabulary

Synonyms (similar to) – impatience, annoyance, displeasure, resentment, exasperation, fury, rage, wrath, outrage

Antonyms (opposite of) – calmness, agreeability, contentment, happiness, joy, peace, pleasantness

---

Anxiety

Anxiety is an unpleasant feeling that makes you feel uneasy, afraid, or worried about something – real or imagined. It is also a mood you can have for a long period of time that is not always related to something that is happening right in front of you. People are usually anxious about unpleasant things that they feel they won't be able to control or avoid.

Think back to the story about Tessa in the beginning of this chapter. Tessa's fear of "characters" did not happen only when she saw them. Just the suggestion that she *might* see one caused her a lot of anxiety in the long term. That's probably why she became so upset when her family talked about going to Disney World.

Anxiety is a normal reaction to stress, or a difficult situation at home or at school. Too much anxiety or worry for a long period of time, or worries about things that aren't likely to happen, can be very difficult to manage by oneself. Although Tessa was anxious about characters for a long period of time, it seemed that she really only thought about it when her family talked about it or when she knew she was going to be in a situation where she would see them. However, if Tessa started to become anxious about running into a "character" at school and it started affecting her ability to get up and go to school, she would probably need to get some help from a counselor or therapist.

When you are experiencing anxiety, you might feel the following kinds of physical sensations throughout your body:

- A quicker heartbeat
- Flushed, or red, in the face
- Sweaty palms
- Shaky legs or body – weak muscles
- Stomachache, nausea
- Difficulty breathing, chest pain
- Headaches

Not everyone feels all of these things at once, and some might never feel any of them. **Remember emotions are very different for everyone.**

When you look at someone who is feeling nervous, you might see that their face has turned pale, they might be shaking or sweating, and their pupils may have grown larger. You may have the same reactions when you feel nervous.

Here are some sentences with words that describe "levels" or "degrees" of anxiety:

Uneasiness: Relates to being uncomfortable, restless, or disturbed: "Sydney has feelings of **uneasiness** before she meets new people, but they usually go away quickly."

Concern: Relates to something that affects a person's welfare or happiness: "I have some news about changes in our school that really **concern** me."

Panic: Relates to a sudden overwhelming fear that produces irrational behavior: "Sara began to **panic** once she realized that she was late for her flight."

 # Quick Review

What Is Anxiety?

- An unpleasant feeling of being uneasy, afraid or worried

- Can be a normal reaction to feeling stress

- Can be caused by something real or something in your imagination

How Does Anxiety Feel?

- Rapid heartbeat

- Difficulty breathing, chest pain

- Sweaty palms

- Flushed or pale in the face

- Shaky, jittery legs, hands, fingers

- Headaches

- Nausea

Body Language and Facial Expression Clues for Anxiety

The clues depend on the intensity of the anxiety. Less intense anxiety can sometimes look like sadness and more intense (very big) anxiety can look like fear. You will need to use other clues about the context to help you.

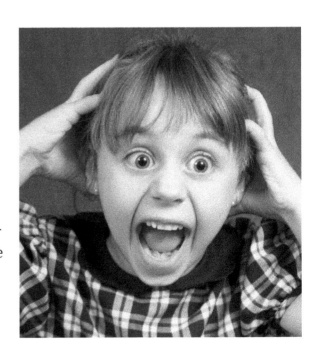

- Pale face

- Shaking, sweating

- Raised brow – pulled toward the center of the forehead, eyebrows straight

- Open eyes

- Possibly an open or outstretched mouth or teeth clenched

Anxiety Vocabulary

Synonyms (similar to) – nervous, worried, concerned, distressed, edgy, jittery, jumpy, uneasy, worried, troubled, panicked, dread, apprehensive

Antonyms (opposite of) – calm, cool, collected, relaxed

Boredom

Boredom is an unpleasant feeling, usually in response to an experience or activity that is dull, uninteresting, or for some reason difficult to concentrate on. Everyone feels bored with things at one time or another. Sometimes it is hard to tell if you are bored. But you are probably feeling bored if you are feeling like you can't pay attention to something you have been doing for a long time, or if you are wishing that you were doing something different.

It is also possible that you could feel bored when you are with a friend doing something together that you don't really want to do. For example, maybe you have a friend who loves to watch soccer on TV. You don't know much about soccer and don't care to watch soccer games. You prefer to watch golf, because that's what really interests you. Suppose your friend invites you over to hang out. When you get to his house, he wants you to come into the living room where he is watching a soccer match. Since you want to spend time with him, you try to pay attention to the game, but before long, you are restless and need a change because you are feeling bored.

Sometimes you can feel bored when you have to pay attention to something for a long time, like when you are in school, a place of worship, or having to do things your parents or other adults want you to do. At these times, you may even feel like you are being "forced" to do something you don't want to do. Everyone feels bored some of the time, and everyone has a different idea of what is boring. It's what you do in response to your feelings of boredom that is important.

Being bored is sometimes a positive thing, because it can motivate you to find something exciting to do. For example, when you are feeling bored at home, you might become motivated to call a friend to see if she wants to go to a movie with you. When you are alone, you might find things to do that will help you get through the boredom, like reading a book, watching TV, or finding a friend to hang out with.

But being bored can also cause problems if you aren't careful. It is easy to become distracted when you are bored, which can lead to doing things that might interrupt or upset others. For example, suppose you are in class listening to the teacher talk about a book that you've already read and decided you don't like. You might become less interested in listening and start focusing on something else to fight the boredom, like doodling on paper, cleaning out your desk, or talking to somebody sitting next to you. When your teacher notices that you aren't paying attention, you might get into trouble.

You can express your feelings when you are bored, as long as you do it in a polite way. If you feel bored when a friend has chosen an activity that you aren't interested in, nicely suggest something else to do. Share your opinion, but don't make your friend feel bad for having different interests than you. In the example above where your friend wants to watch soccer and you don't, you might say something like, "I don't feel like watching soccer right now, do you think we could talk about doing something different?"

If you feel bored when you are at school, or during an activity that an adult wants you to do, be sure to express your feelings at an appropriate time – not in the middle of the activity. For example, interrupting your teacher during class to say, "I hated this book, this is so boring," shows that you are not thinking about what the other people around you are thinking and feeling. But talking with your teacher about your feelings after the class is over might help you solve your problem.

Here are some sentences with words that describe "levels" or "degrees" of boredom:

Uninterested: Describes not being interested in something: "Young children are often **uninterested** in adult conversations."

Dull: Refers to something that is boring: "I couldn't believe how **dull** that assembly was, I almost fell asleep."

Monotonous: Uninteresting or boring as a result of being repetitive or unchanging: "It wasn't the singer that made me hate that song, it was just that **monotonous** beat."

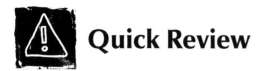 **Quick Review**

What Is Boredom?

- A response or feeling to something dull or uninteresting

What Does Boredom Feel Like?

- Tiredness or difficulty staying awake

- Slow movements

Body Language and Facial Expression Clues for Boredom

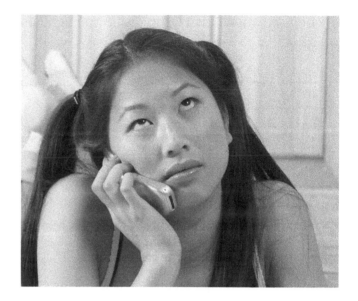

The clues for boredom might be:

- Not paying attention

- Head-resting-in-hands posture

- Eyes closing or looking sleepy

- Moving away or trying to move away from what is boring.

Boredom Vocabulary

Synonyms (similar to) – weariness, apathy, lethargy, listlessness, unconcern, uninterested, detachment, indifference, monotonous, dullness

Antonyms (opposite of) – interested, captivated, excited, exhilarated, thrilled

---

Embarrassment

Embarrassment is an experience you might have when your thoughts or actions that are not socially acceptable are revealed to or witnessed by other people. You may feel some loss of "dignity" or "honor" depending on the situation. In other words, embarrassment is a feeling you have when you do or say something in front of other people that is unexpected and that might make you feel bad about yourself in some way.

When you are embarrassed, you might feel your face getting warm. It might turn red or "flushed." You may have the feeling that "everyone is looking at you or staring, and you may be "flustered" or confused about what to do next. You might also feel as if you want to leave the scene as soon as possible.

Everyone feels embarrassed some time. Common social situations where you might feel embarrassed include:

- Dropping your lunch tray in the lunchroom at school
- Saying the "wrong thing" in front of friends, like mispronouncing or forgetting somebody's name
- Unintentionally hurting someone's feelings
- Giving the wrong answer in class
- Tripping while walking in front of other people
- If someone you know finds out that you were saying unkind things about them

Being embarrassed also has a lot to do with what you *think* other people are thinking about you. For example, you might feel embarrassed if you try to do something and fail while others are watching. You feel embarrassed because you know that others are watching and thinking about your mistake. You might feel that since they have seen the mistake, they might be thinking badly about you.

Here are sentences with words that describe "levels" or "degrees" of embarrassment:

Flustered: Describes feeling disturbed, troubled, or disoriented: "She immediately became **flustered** when the teacher unexpectedly asked her to read her homework assignment in front of the class."

Foolish: Describes feeling silly, immature, or even idiotic: "Even though Nancy loved drama class, she still felt **foolish** doing some of the activities in front of her friends."

Ashamed: Describes feeling remorseful or regretful about something occurring in a social situation: "Charles really felt **ashamed** when everyone at school found out that he was the one who had stolen the answers to the English test."

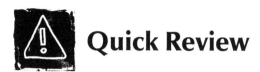 **Quick Review**

What Is Embarrassment?

- Feeling like others have seen or heard that you have done something that is not socially acceptable

- Making a mistake in front of other people and feeling bad about it

How Does Embarrassed Feel?

- Blushing or flushed cheeks

- Shaky, jittery legs, hands, fingers like nervousness

Body Language and Facial Expression Clues for Embarrassment

A person who is feeling embarrassed may look a lot like someone who is nervous or surprised.

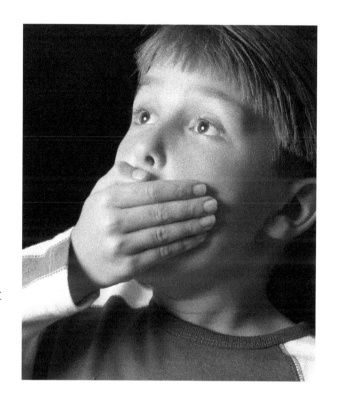

Embarrassment Vocabulary

Synonyms (similar to) – humiliated, ashamed, self-conscious, uneasy, awkward, uncomfortable, flustered, foolish

Antonyms (opposite of) – calm, certain, confident, at ease, proud, reassured, relaxed, comfortable, agreeable

Disappointment

Disappointment refers to an experience of being "let down." You may feel disappointed if you are expecting that something will be a certain way and someone or something prevents it from happening that way. For example:

- Your plans to go to a movie with a friend get canceled because your friend is feeling sick.

- You are excited to get your favorite ice cream, but when you get to the store, they are out of the flavor you wanted.

- Your baseball team lost an important baseball game.

When you are disappointed, you might also feel angry, sad, or annoyed. You might feel like saying or doing mean things to others or yourself, but this is not the appropriate way to handle things. Disappointments happen. If you are not prepared for them, you may find yourself feeling sad for long periods of time, and this can be very stressful.

To avoid that from happening, thinking about your actions and reactions to disappointment is helpful. You can also try some of these ideas to help you make choices that are more socially acceptable:

- Express your feelings of disappointment to someone who has the time to listen attentively to you. Explain to them why you are feeling disappointed.

- If you were disappointed because of something a friend did or didn't do, try to find out from them what happened. You don't want to be angry with someone who canceled your plan to go to the movies because she had to stay home because she was sick. It's not her fault that she got sick.

- Make a plan for how things will be different for you in the future. This includes how you might deal with future disappointments that are similar, or how you might react or communicate with others.

Here are sentences with words that describe "levels" or "degrees" of disappointment:

Dissatisfaction: Describes a feeling of discontent or unhappiness: "My teacher expressed her **dissatisfaction** with my final project by giving me a really bad grade."

Distress: Describes a feeling of having "bad luck" in a situation: "Whenever my team loses an important game, I leave with a feeling of great **distress.**"

Frustration: Describes feeling great disappointment or having been prevented from doing something: "My feelings of **frustration** kept getting worse when I left messages for my boyfriend over the weekend and he wouldn't return my calls."

 # Quick Review

What Is Disappointed?

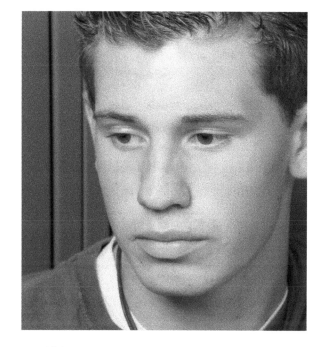

- Feeling like you have been "let down" by someone or something

- Expecting that something will happen that doesn't

How Does Disappointed Feel?

- A little bit of angry, a little bit of sad … it's a difficult feeling

- It may make you feel like you want to distract yourself from the feeling or get angry at someone

Body Language and Facial Expression Clues for Disappointed

A person who is feeling disappointed may look a lot like someone who is feeling sad.

Disappointment Vocabulary

Synonyms (similar to) – cheated, dissatisfied, let down, failed, distressed, frustrated

Antonyms (opposite of) – satisfied, fulfilled

Disgust

Disgust describes a feeling of dislike that is very strong. In fact, it may be so strong that it can make your stomach upset or queasy. You might have an experience of seeing something that you think is "gross" and then want to remove yourself from the situation. In this example, you could say that you are feeling disgusted, as in: "I was so disgusted by that frog dissection in biology class that I had to leave the room."

You can also use disgust to describe feeling repelled or offended by someone's behavior. For example, "Eating with people who chew with their mouth open is disgusting."

What makes somebody feel disgusted is very different for everyone. Something that might disgust you might not affect someone else in the same way. For example, you might not want to watch certain kinds of movies or TV shows because they include violent or gruesome scenes, but maybe your best friend loves that stuff. Deciding what to watch when you are together could be challenging, but not if you are able to consider each other's point of view.

Here are some sentences with words that describe "levels" or "degrees" of disgust:

Objection: Describes a feeling of disagreement with someone or something: "My mother has an **objection** to having boys and girls hanging out in our house when there is no adult home."

Loathing: Describes an intense feeling of dislike: "Melissa's **loathing** of Indian food prevented us from going to that new restaurant in the city."

Revulsion: Describes a strong feeling of disgust or hatred toward something: "My camp counselors tried their best, but they could not change the feelings of **revulsion** I had about walking through that smelly, swampy bog."

 Quick Review

What Is Disgust?

- A very strong feeling of dislike
- Usually associated with things that are not clean, not edible, or unhealthy

How Does Disgust Feel?

- Can be emotional disgust, where you feel irritated or annoyed by someone's behavior

- Can be physical disgust, making you feel sick to your stomach

Body Language and Facial Expression Clues for Disgust

- Mostly seen on the face around the nose and the mouth

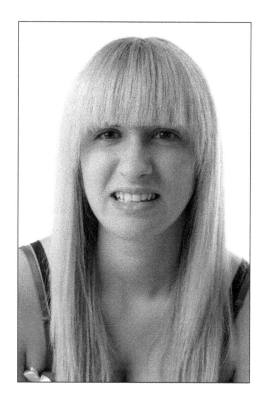

Physical Disgust (directed toward a thing):

- Person may look like she is about ready to vomit or stick her tongue out in an exaggerated way

- Mouth is open, with or without the tongue sticking out.

- Eyes are narrowed or squeezed shut

- Head turned away from the thing that is disgusting

- Raised or flared nostrils

- Bridge of the nose crinkled – eyes and the area around the eyes move toward that area of the face

Emotional Disgust (directed toward a person):

- Smile may be more like a "sneer" or asymmetrical (not even)

- Relaxed lower lip and mouth that is closed or only slightly open

---

Disgust Vocabulary

Synonyms (similar to) – nauseated, repulsed, sickened, turned off, repelled, grossed out, loathed, revulsion

Antonyms (opposite of) – prefer, fond of, like, attracted, delighted

---

Envy

Envy is a word that describes when you are feeling like you don't have something that someone else has or does, and you want it. This can be a character trait (like being smart or having a lot of friends), a possession (like owning the newest computer or having expensive clothes), or an achievement (like being the captain of a winning sports team, making the honor roll, or even having a serious boyfriend or girlfriend) that the other person has and that you would really like for yourself.

Envy can be painful, as your desire for that something or somebody that another person has may make you wish that the other person would lose those great qualities, possessions, or achievements. You may feel resentful toward that person, even if it is someone that you are very close with, and this can make a relationship difficult.

For example, suppose you have a friend who wears expensive, trendy clothes to school every day. You might be someone who likes to dress nicely and in style, yet buying expensive clothing isn't something that you and your family can afford on a regular basis. Maybe you have great outfits, but they aren't necessarily the pricey designer-label ones that your friend wears. If you are spending a lot of time thinking about how much you would like your friend's wardrobe, or even wishing that your friend wasn't able to have such neat clothes, you are probably feeling envious.

It may be hard for you to keep envious feelings to yourself. You might act and or say things that will give others clues about how you are feeling, and this can sometimes change their opinion of you. Sometimes you might not even realize that you are showing these feelings to others.

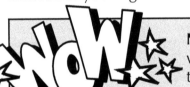

NOTE: **Jealousy** is word that people sometimes use interchangeably with **envy**. They are similar terms, but they describe different emotional states.

Jealousy is a fear of losing something you have to another person. Usually, this is about a loved one like a friend, often a boyfriend or girlfriend. **Envy** is a feeling of pain or frustration caused by another person having something that you don't have. Envy usually involves two people (you can be envious of more than one person at a time), and jealousy usually involves three people. You might feel jealous when your best friend starts hanging out with someone else more than you, because you are afraid that they might enjoy the other person more, and stop being friendly with you.

Here are some sentences with words that describe "levels" or "degrees" of envy:

Yearning: Describes a strong desire or hope for something: "Reina's **yearning** to do well in her science class grew stronger when her best friend Jamie did better than her on the exam."

Resentment: Describes feeling or wishing that someone did not have something that you want: "Nancy couldn't control her feelings of **resentment** toward Faith for getting the lead in the school musical."

Rivalry: Describes feelings of envy that occur on a continuous basis: "Mindy's constant bragging about her musical ability created a huge **rivalry** between her and the other clarinet players in the band."

 # Quick Review

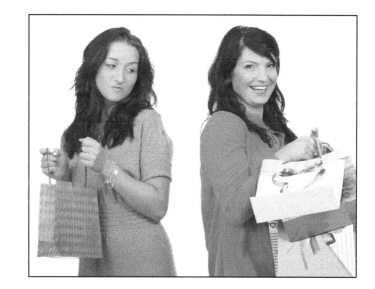

What Is Envy?

- A strong feeling of wanting something that someone else has or can do

How Does Envy Feel?

- Feeling envious can affect your self-esteem or make you feel "not good enough"

- It feels a lot like unhappiness or sometimes anger toward a person you are envious of

Body Language and Facial Expression Clues for Envy

- Eyes staring

- Corners of the mouth turned down, may look like a "sneer"

- Chin jutting out

Envy Vocabulary

Synonyms (similar to) – jealousy, resentment, rivalry, yearning, competitiveness, covetousness, animosity

Antonyms (opposite of) – kindness, goodwill, comfort, confidence

---

Fear

When you experience fear, you are generally expecting, or aware of, "danger." Fear is a response to something that you know is real. For example, when you are on your way to the doctor for an exam and know that you will have to get a shot or some other procedure that will cause you pain, you might feel afraid.

Fear is different than anxiety. When you worry on a regular basis about getting shots at the doctor, even when it is not happening any time soon, you are probably feeling anxiety.

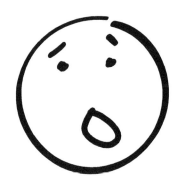

Your body is built to help you deal with feeling fear. It gets ready to protect itself immediately when you are feeling afraid. Some of the things that happen to you physically when you are afraid include:

- Tightened muscles

- Increased body temperature and perspiration

- Increased heart rate and heart beat

- Physical movements like "covering" parts of the body to protect them, or even "jumping" or moving away from the thing that is frightening

Many words are used to describe the experience of fear. People may use these terms interchangeably, but there are differences in their meanings, usually to specify degree or level of fear.

Here are sentences with words that describe "levels" or "degrees" of fear:

Dread: Suggests being unwilling to face something: "I **dread** hearing bad news over the telephone" or "I am **dreading** getting my test back because I know I didn't do well."

Alarm: Describes an experience of strong emotional upset caused by unexpected or immediate danger: "I was **alarmed** by the smell of smoke in the hallway" or "The sound of the fireworks was extremely loud and **alarming**."

Fright: Refers to the shock of something startling, and suggests a brief experience: "I felt **frightened** right as the plane took off, but I calmed down once we were in the air," or "I don't like it when you come into my room without knocking first; it really **frightens** me."

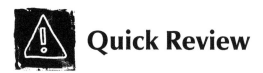

Quick Review

What Is Fear?

- Feeling scared or frightened of a danger that is real or imagined

How Does Fear Feel?

- It is generally not a lasting feeling

- It's an uncomfortable feeling

- Makes people want to run away from the thing that is making them afraid

Body Language and Facial Expression Clues for Fear

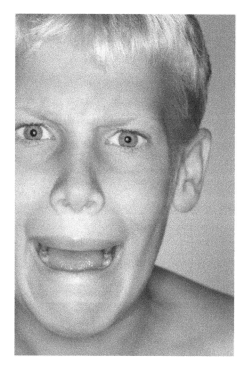

- Tense muscles

- Increased breathing and heart rate

- Shaking

- Raised eyebrows – different from surprise, because the eyebrows are pulled toward the center of the forehead in fear

- Eyebrows are less arched and straighter than surprise

- Open eyes

- Open, stretched mouth

Fear Vocabulary

Synonyms (similar to) – uneasiness, distress, fright, dread, alarm, panic, horror, terror, trepidation, apprehension, agitation

Antonyms (opposite of) – confidence, fearlessness, courageousness, bravery, dauntlessness

---

Frustration

Frustration refers to the experience of trying hard to do something or get something that you want and then not being able to do it or get it. For example, maybe you have wanted to see a certain movie, and every time you ask your mom if she can take you to the movie theater she is not available. You aren't old enough to drive, so you have to wait until someone can drop you off. These are things that are out of your control, but they are "blocking" your goal, and that can make you feel frustrated.

Frustration can be a good thing, as it may motivate you to solve a problem. Like in the example above, maybe you will work hard to search out a different way to get to the movies. Maybe your frustration will make you call every friend you can think of to try to find someone who might be available to go to the movies and whose mother or father can give you a ride. Or, it might make you learn about using public transportation, like taking a bus, if your parents will let you.

Frustration is related to **anger** and **disappointment**. If you are not able to deal with your frustration in a positive way, like finding appropriate solutions to the "obstacles" you face, your frustration may "build" until you are unable to deal with it at all. Or, it may "push" you to make poor choices or even lead to behaviors that can cause more problems. Suppose, in the movie example above, you took your frustration out on your mom by yelling at her and starting a big argument. Or, maybe you looked to find something else to do like watching TV and then got in a huge fight with your sister or brother over what to watch. Expressing your frustration over one problem in an inappropriate way can cause more problems.

Here are sentences with words that describe "levels" or "degrees" of frustration:

Discouraged: Describes feeling disheartened, fearful, or nervous about something: "I was really **discouraged** to see that no one signed up to help out at the fifth grade car wash fundraiser."

Overwhelmed: Suggests feeling "beaten" by outside factors: "I am so **overwhelmed** by the amount of homework in math this year that I can barely do anything for my other subjects."

Exasperated: Suggests feeling really angry, irritated, or upset by something or someone: "Deborah had become completely **exasperated** and could no longer fight with her mother about extending her curfew to 11:00 pm."

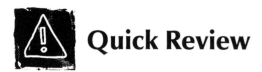 **Quick Review**

What Is Frustration?

- Trying to do something or get something you really want and then not being able to do it, or get it

How Does Frustration Feel?

- Like you are being prevented from doing something that you really want to do

- Related to anger and disappointment

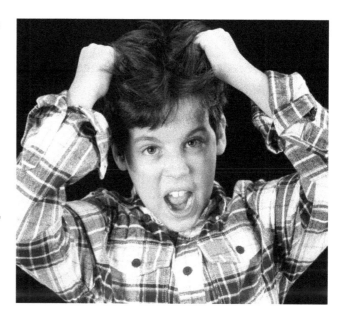

Body Language and Facial Expression Clues for Frustration

- Similar to anger or possibly disgust

- Red or flushed face

- Clenched fists

Frustration Vocabulary

Synonyms (similar to) – annoyed, let down, discouraged, disheartened, irritated, foiled, overwhelmed, defeated, exasperated, disappointed, failed, dissatisfied

Antonyms (opposite of) – calm, at ease, happy, joyful, successful, content, satisfied

---

Pride

Feeling pride (proud) means that you are feeling happy or excited about something special that you have done.

Getting a good grade, winning a game, finishing a project, and doing better than the last time on something that was hard for you are different reasons you might feel proud. Pride can happen when others or when you yourself recognize what a great job you have done and you receive praise for it.

Pride is different than happiness because it has to do with sharing your "accomplishments" with others, either verbally or nonverbally. When you feel proud of yourself, you might show it by lifting your chin, smiling, or placing your hands on your hips to indicate confidence or demonstrate victory. You may also choose to tell someone about what is making you feel proud.

It's good to let others know when you are feeling proud of something you have accomplished. Your close friends and family will definitely be interested in hearing about these things. Since you have close relationships with them, it will probably make them feel proud and happy for you. That will make you feel proud and happy also.

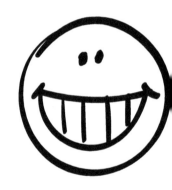

However, telling others about something you have done well can be tricky. Whoever you speak with should understand that you are sharing information that is important to you and that you are not being boastful. Being boastful is like bragging. It means that you are talking about yourself too much and with too much pride. Nobody wants to listen to somebody talking too much about themselves, and talking about how great your accomplishments are can make others feel less confident or even annoyed, especially when they are hearing the same things over and over again. So, **no bragging and no repeating the same things over and over.**

Definitely tell others when you have done something special or important, especially when it is something that you think they will feel excited about also. For example, if you've studied really hard for a test and got an "A," this would be something important to share with close friends or family members, but it might not be a great thing to share with other kids in your class who didn't do as well.

Here are some sentences with words that describe "levels" or "degrees" of pride:

Confident: Suggests feeling positive about something: "Risa felt **confident** that she was ready for the performance."

Proud: Suggests having positive feelings about one's own conduct, or someone else's: "Kristen wasn't sure that she had done very well at cheerleading try-outs, but she was **proud** of herself for trying."

Self-worth: Suggests understanding one's own positive characteristics: "Although Monica usually had very positive feelings of **self-worth,** she couldn't manage being teased by Rebecca at lunch.

 Quick Review

What Is Pride?

- Feeling happy or excited about something special you have done

- Feeling great about an accomplishment

How Does Pride Feel?

- It's a lot like happiness or excitement

- Like you want to share your feelings with others

Body Language and Facial Expression Clues for Pride

- Similar to happiness

- Mouth smiling and either open or closed

- Eyes "squinted" due to big smile

- Body position demonstrating "victory," hands on hips, high five, or other gestures

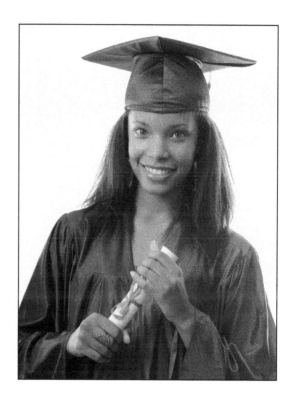

Pride Vocabulary

Synonyms (similar to) – self-assured, confident, self-satisfied, self-esteem, dignity

Antonyms (opposite to) – humble, modest, unpretentious, humility

---

Big Picture Thinking and Feelings and Emotions

Your thoughts about a situation that you are in bring about feelings. You understand how you are feeling by labeling the feeling with an emotion word.

Your thoughts and feelings guide your actions and reactions in different situations. For example, when you are feeling happy, you probably look happy to others and behave in a way that shows others that you are feeling good, like being more helpful or talkative. On the other hand, if you are feeling unhappy, you probably look unhappy to others and behave in a way that shows others that you are not feeling good about things.

Remember to pay close attention to your feelings when you are socializing. Understanding your emotions will help you better understand yourself. It will also help you better understand what other people might be thinking and feeling when you are with them.

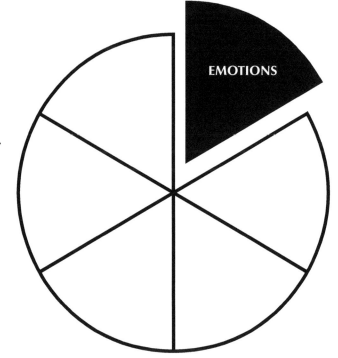

 KIDS IN ACTION REVIEW

Thinking back to the story example at the beginning of this chapter, you can see that the way Tessa responded to her fear was affecting both herself and her family. Without Tessa identifying and expressing the feelings she was having, neither she nor her family would have known how to move forward and solve the conflict. In the end, they might have decided to stay home to everybody's disappointment. Instead, once Tessa started to explain her feelings using emotion words, they were able to start coming up with solutions for how to deal with the problem, so they could have a great vacation after all.

Understanding feelings and emotions can help you make better choices about how to act, or react, in a situation, which is helpful to us when we want to solve problems that happen when we are in social situations. The act of trying to solve those kinds of problems is sometimes referred to as **social problem solving.**

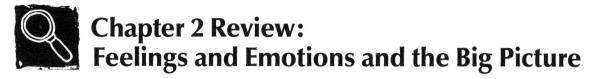

Chapter 2 Review: Feelings and Emotions and the Big Picture

In this chapter, we talked about how important it is to think about feelings and emotions. You need to be able to understand your emotions and the emotions of others in order to be socially successful. Social situations bring about different feelings for everyone involved. Understanding your own and others' emotions is an important part of being able to see the Big Picture in social situations.

Practice Ideas

1. **Emotions Dictionary.** Make a "dictionary" of emotion words. Use the basic emotions listed in this chapter as a guide and then see if you can add more vocabulary words.

2. **Emotions Thesaurus.** Make a "thesaurus" of emotion words. Use the synonyms and antonyms listed on the emotion pages to help you and then see if you can add more.

3. **Interactive Emotions Reference.** Make your "dictionary" and "thesaurus" interactive. Add pictures to show the feelings that are highlighted. These can be photographs, pictures from magazines or books, or downloaded and printed from the Internet.

4. **"Special Times" Scrapbook.** Go through family photos and find pictures of you experiencing different emotions. Even though you might be "smiling" in some of the photos, think back to where you were and what you were doing at the time and focus on how you were feeling. Make scrapbook pages of the photographs and label the page with the emotion you were feeling. Write a short description on the page of what was happening and how you were feeling at the time.

5. **What's Happening.** Cut out pictures of people experiencing different emotions from magazines or find them on the Internet. Glue the pictures onto one side of an index card. On the other side, try to think of a situation that the person in the picture could be involved in that might be causing him or her to feel that particular emotion. Go further:
   • Once you have thought of a situation for each card, go back through them and try to come up with a different possibility.
   • Share your ideas with a partner, and see if they can come up with a different situation.

6. **Name and Number.** Once you have reviewed the emotion words in this chapter, start to use them in your everyday life. Stop yourself periodically and think about what you are feeling – use the Feeling Thermometer if you wish. Give that feeling an emotion word so that you have a better understanding of what is happening for you. Go further with this and also give the emotion a number, from 1 to 10 (10 being the most or worst and 1 being the least) as you are experiencing

it. Check in with yourself after 5 minutes and give the emotion a number again. Did the number change? Did it go down or up?

You can also use the Incredible 5-Point Scale (you can find a blank one in the Appendix on page A5) to help you think about degrees of emotion in the same way. See how you're feeling, give the feeling an emotion word, and locate where you are on the scale. Then check in with yourself and see if the number changed.

7. **Emotions Record.** Find examples in your life of the emotions discussed in this chapter. Pick an emotion and list times when you have observed yourself or someone else feeling that way. Think about what it "felt" like for you physically and what it "looked" like to you and to the other people around you. How did you and the others around you know what feeling you were experiencing? Make a note if you think you need to act or react differently next time. The following is an example you can use as a guide and there is a blank one in the Appendix on page A7.

Situation	Emotion	What It Felt Like	What It Looked Like	Did I Express Myself to Others Appropriately?
Asked my parents for permission to go to the movies with a friend. They said no because we had other family plans.	Angry, frustrated	I felt really angry, and it was hard for me to tolerate the level of frustration I had from dealing with their "NO" answer.	I acted out of control, had a tantrum with a lot of crying and door slamming and yelling.	No. I should have been able to handle my anger better.

8. **Emotions Line-Up.** Rank order emotion words and their synonyms by how intense you perceive them to be. For example, *angry, irate, furious, mad, outraged,* and *displeased* all describe the same emotion family, but what kind of "mad" do you picture when you hear each word? Put them in order from highest to lowest (REALLY MAD to slightly irritated).

9. **Feeling Thermometer.** Choose a situation that you have experienced or one that someone else has experienced, and get a copy of the blank Feeling Thermometer in the Appendix on page A4. Use the Feeling Thermometer to represent how you, or the other person, experienced a particular emotion during that situation. For example, suppose you want to take another look at how you handled an argument with a close friend. Maybe you were fighting about what movie to see, and you had a hard time accepting your friend's thoughts and opinions on this topic. Maybe you were feeling angry with your friend and frustrated because he wouldn't listen to you when you told him that all the reviews on the Internet said that the movie he had picked was really bad, and he wanted to see it anyway. You could label your thermometer "Frustrated" and number the levels from 1 to 10, 10 being the highest level of frustration and 1 being the lowest. Figure out your level and fill in the thermometer up to your level.

After you have filled in the thermometer, label the Feeling Thermometer numbers 1–10 with words from the emotion family to describe "how high" or "how low" your emotional reaction was. In the example above about frustration, you might give number 1 the word "bothered," and number 10 something like "exasperated" because the word describes a huge amount of frustration.

10. **5-Point Scale for Emotions.** Make a copy of the 5-Point Scale that is included in the Appendix on page A7. Complete a scale for each of the basic emotions: **sadness, happiness, disgust, anger, fear and surprise**. For example, you might represent anger/fear like this:

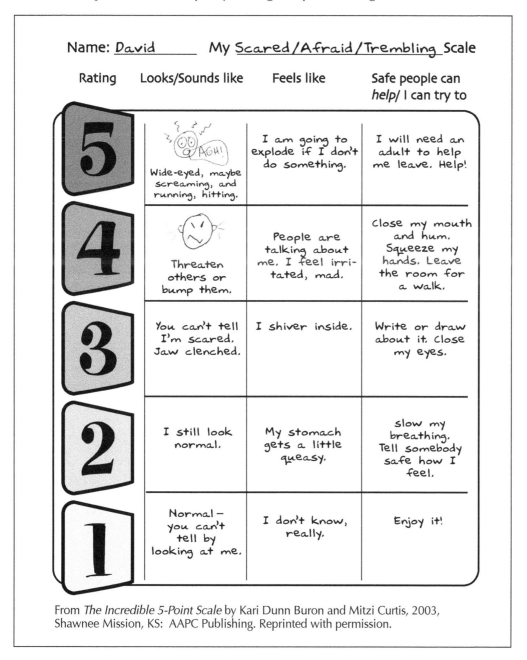

Name: David   My Scared/Afraid/Trembling Scale

Rating	Looks/Sounds like	Feels like	Safe people can *help*/ I can try to
5	Wide-eyed, maybe screaming, and running, hitting.	I am going to explode if I don't do something.	I will need an adult to help me leave. Help!
4	Threaten others or bump them.	People are talking about me. I feel irritated, mad.	Close my mouth and hum. Squeeze my hands. Leave the room for a walk.
3	You can't tell I'm scared. Jaw clenched.	I shiver inside.	Write or draw about it. Close my eyes.
2	I still look normal.	My stomach gets a little queasy.	slow my breathing. Tell somebody safe how I feel.
1	Normal — you can't tell by looking at me.	I don't know, really.	Enjoy it!

From *The Incredible 5-Point Scale* by Kari Dunn Buron and Mitzi Curtis, 2003, Shawnee Mission, KS: AAPC Publishing. Reprinted with permission.

After completing the charts for the basic emotions, keep them handy in your journal or notebook so that you can refer back to them as needed.

11. **Journal Entries.** Keep an emotions journal. Entries might include the following:
    - Date of the event you want to analyze
    - Description of the situation – who, what, when, where, etc.
    - The feelings you experienced
    - A description of the emotions you think others may have been feeling
    - Some thoughts about whether the emotions you experienced were appropriate for the situation (for example, were they "too much" or "too little"?)
    - A description of the outcome of the situation or what you might have learned from it

12. **Be an Actor.** Use a mirror or perform for someone else. See if you can pantomime what a particular emotion might look like.

13. **Emotion Charades.** Play Emotion Charades with a partner. List as many emotions as you can on slips of paper and then throw them into a bowl. Choose someone to go first and be the "actor." The person selects a slip of paper from the bowl, reads the emotion, and keeps it to him/herself. Then the actor performs the emotion in the following ways:
    - Using facial expressions, body language and words (easier)
    - Using just facial expressions and body language and no words (harder)

    It is the job of the "guesser" to determine what kind of emotion is being displayed.

14. **TV and Movies.** Watch a TV show or movie with an adult who is working with you. Analyze the characters and their emotions as they occur in relation to the different situations that they dealt with in the show. Here are some questions to guide you:
    - Did the character (or characters) encounter any problems? What were they?
    - What emotions did you observe the characters experience before the problem occurred? What were they feeling after the problem occurred?
    - How did the character solve the problem?
    - What did the character seem to be feeling after the problem was solved?

Chapter 3

The Big Picture: Self-Control

This chapter discusses **self-control**. Expressing your thoughts and feelings is important, but you need to do so in a way that will help you and not distract other people or yourself.

Self-control means keeping your thoughts, emotions, and physical activity to yourself until you can make a good decision about how to express them. Self-control means exactly what it says, being in "control" of everything about "yourself." Sometimes people use other words to describe being in control of ourselves, such as "composure," "self-regulation," "modulation," or "self-restraint." These are just different words that mean pretty much the same thing. What people want and need you to be thinking about is how you are keeping your behavior, thoughts, and emotions "in check."

 KIDS IN ACTION: SELF-CONTROL

Evan is a fifth grader who is very active. He plays soccer and ice hockey and enjoys playing sports during recess and gym when he is in school. He prefers to be outside running, rather than inside sitting still. He is a kid who is "in motion" a lot. Even when he is not playing sports, he is thinking or talking with his friends about them.

Evan is very smart and learns things easily, but it can be difficult for him to pay attention in class. His activity level is high, and sometimes it is difficult for him to stay in his seat quietly and not call out answers when he knows them. Other kids, things around the classroom, and his own thoughts about what he will be doing after school easily distract him. Sometimes he finishes his work much quicker than the other students in his class and has trouble finding appropriate things to do with his extra time.

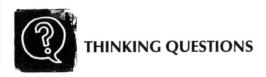 **THINKING QUESTIONS**

What is Evan's problem?

Why do you think that Evan's behavior is a problem for the people around him?

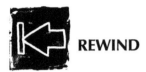 **REWIND**

Evan needs to be able to adjust his behavior to the situation that he is in. He can't bring his "high" level of activity into the classroom, and he must be able to regulate, or **adjust the time, amount, degree, or rate** of his behavior so that it is appropriate for the classroom.

Understanding self-control is important because you need to be able to:
- Keep calm when you are experiencing difficult emotions and express them in an appropriate way that will help you effectively communicate your wants and needs.
- Express both positive and negative feelings in a way that is appropriate for where you are and who you are with. This shows that you are considering the people around you and matching your reactions to the situation.
- Mind your manners when you are interacting with others.
- Change the types of manners that you use when you are in different situations.
- Deal with distractions!
- Make sure you are not impulsive – both verbally and/or physically.
- Stay calm and focused when you are facing changes that sometimes arise in your life.
- Limit the amount of arguing you do with others.
- Keep your body from moving around too much and invading other people's space.

This is a long list of things that you need to think about all the time. These things are important to remember because your behavior "says" something about you to the other people around you.

This chapter will help you to better understand self-control, and it will also give you some ideas about situations where you need to exercise self-control and how to exercise better self-control when you need to. You will read about:
- What behaviors are appropriate at home and at school
- What behaviors are considered inappropriate at home and at school
- Flexible and inflexible thinking
- Dealing with difficult emotions

- Common ways people try to get calm and stay calm
- Self-talk strategies
- How to ignore distractions and other things

Self-control is an important part of interacting with others. Your behavior has an effect on the people who are near you, whether you know them or not, and that can affect how they think about you. Your goal should be to keep them thinking about you in a positive way. When people think about you in a positive way, they will be more interested in communicating and interacting with you. Remember, you always need to interact and communicate with people in order to get the things that you want and need from the world around you. If you look at the illustration below, you can see how the cycle works:

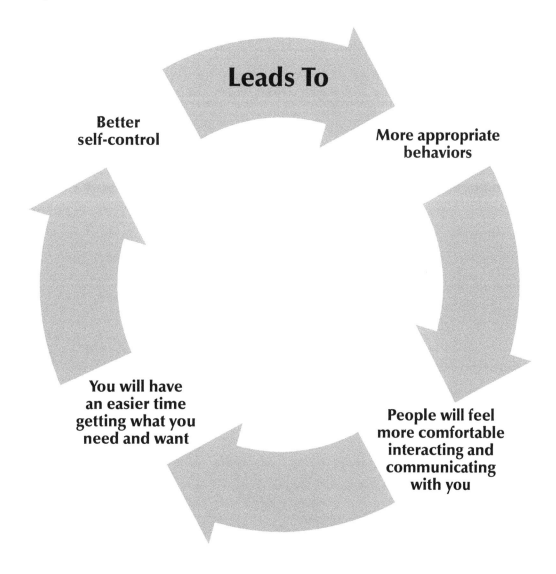

Appropriate and Inappropriate Behaviors

Certain situations call for certain kinds of behavior. For example, in school you need to follow the rules and pay attention. When you are in a restaurant, you need to use good manners and respect other diners.

Sometimes, when adults want to remind you to think about your behavior, they sometimes use the words *appropriate* or *inappropriate*. For example, you are having dinner at a restaurant with your family, and you raise your voice to an uncomfortable level. Your mom might say something like, "Robert, your voice is too loud; it's really inappropriate for a restaurant." **In any situation, *appropriate behavior* means you are following the rules and thinking about self-control, and *inappropriate behavior* means you are not following the rules and not thinking about self-control.**

When you do something that is inappropriate for a particular situation, others might be surprised and even become upset about it. For example, many classrooms have rules about raising your hand instead of blurting out when you want to answer a question. That way, the classroom stays quiet, the teacher knows who wants to participate, and everyone gets a turn. If you shout out an answer without raising your hand, your teacher and the other students in your class will be surprised and perhaps irritated that you were not able to respect the classroom rules in the same way as everyone else.

You need to remember to think about what other people might think about you and your behavior. Doing what is appropriate for a certain situation shows that you are respectful of the rules and thinking of other people. It also shows that you are aware of how important it is to change your behavior in response to the feelings and needs of others. As we said at the beginning of the chapter, people who think positively about you and your behavior are more likely to help you with the things that you want and need.

Sometimes people want to do the opposite of what is appropriate for a situation. For example, maybe a friend in your math class wants to talk out loud to you at a time when the teacher wants you to be working quietly. You might feel you have to respond to your friend, even though you know it's not the right thing to do. This is a time where you need to demonstrate some "self-control" and ignore the distractions around you.

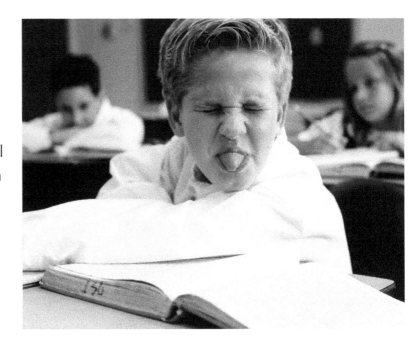

What Is Considered Appropriate Behavior for the Classroom?

Teachers and other students have expectations for you in the classroom. An expectation is a standard of behavior that is required of someone in a specific situation. It is important to match your behaviors to the expectations of others in different situations.

- **Keep your body and eyes on what you are doing.** If you are listening to the teacher talking, that's where your body should be facing and your eyes should be looking. If you are working in a small group with other students, then that's where your body and eyes should be focused.

- **Keep your comments on the topic.** Most teachers expect that students will raise their hand if they want to speak in class, but it is also important that their comments be about the topic at hand. Comments that are not related to the topic should be made after class, for example.

- **Try to keep your body still and sit calmly in your chair.** Moving around a lot is distracting to others. Don't distract others from what they are doing. This means no noises or doing anything that might keep other students from getting things done.

- **Keep negative thoughts to yourself, or find appropriate moments to talk to a friend or your teacher about your feelings.** Everyone gets bored in class sometimes, but you don't need to announce it out loud.

These expectations also apply in other situations where you might be sitting and listening to a grownup in a group, such as at a Scout meeting, religious class, or after-school lessons.

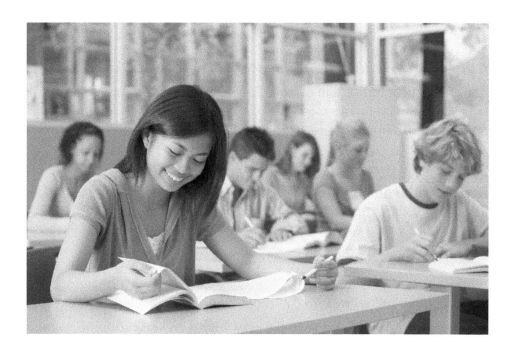

What's Is Considered Inappropriate Behavior for the Classroom?

If you are not doing what is appropriate for the classroom, you might be doing some of these things:

- Wandering away from where you should be
- Distracting other students from what they are doing
- Talking about things that are not related to the topic
- Telling other students what they are doing wrong
- Turning your body and eyes away from others, including the teacher
- Telling people out loud that you are bored
- Calling out answers without raising your hand

Doing things that are not appropriate in the classroom may surprise others, and even upset them. It is distracting, and a teacher will need to take time from teaching to insist that you change your behavior.

What Is Considered Appropriate Behavior at Home?

Home is also a place where you need to exercise self-control. It is easy to forget that family members think about your behavior, but it is important to try to meet their expectations.

Everyone's home life is different, but there are some general statements that can be made to help you understand what's expected at home.

- **Follow the rules.** Whether you like it or not, parents, not children, make the rules. Children can share their thoughts and opinions, but grownups have the final say.

- **Take care of the things you are responsible for, like homework, chores, or your possessions.** Doing these sorts of things will often help you to earn more privileges.

- **Take care of yourself.** It's important for you to keep up with hygiene (grooming, dressing, etc.), nutrition, and exercise.

- **Practice tolerance with your siblings.** This means that you need to be able to deal with what you may consider their "annoying annoyances" without having a meltdown.

- **Be a good host.** If you have a friend over, your parents and siblings will expect that you will be responsible for doing all the things necessary to have a good time with your friend. That means that you are being polite, following rules, and not ignoring your friend's interests or needs. It's not your parent's or your sibling's job to make your friend feel comfortable.

Other important behaviors for home that are considered appropriate:

- Practicing good problem solving

- Communicating honestly with members of your family

- Using good manners

- Being respectful to adults, no matter who they are

You spend a lot of time around your family members, and it can be hard to keep yourself focused all the time. However, try to remember what behavior is appropriate for your home and family.

What Is Considered Inappropriate Behavior at Home?

If you are not doing what is considered appropriate at home, you might be doing some of these things:

- Breaking rules or trying to change them so you can get what you want

- Being irresponsible with your possessions, like losing things, forgetting to put things away, or causing things to break

- Failing to do chores that you are supposed to do to help your family

- Not taking care of your body independently (hygiene, etc.)

- Needing to be reminded to dress appropriately or not spend too much time on the computer

- Fighting too much with your siblings or your parents

- Being disrespectful to adults.

- Not using good manners

- Not being a good host when you have a friend over to your house

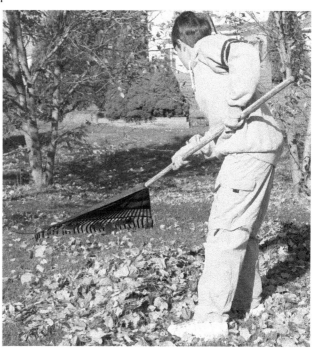

If you do things that are considered inappropriate at home, it can cause difficulty for your family and other people who might be visiting your home, like your parents' friends, a babysitter, or even your own friends. It will upset the people that you have the closest relationships with. Your parents or the adult in charge at home will probably insist that you change your behavior to make everyone feel more comfortable.

Dealing with Difficult Emotions

In Chapter 2, we discussed emotions. Sometimes difficult situations, like a disagreement with a friend or having too much schoolwork to do, can make you feel emotions that are difficult to deal with. "Difficult" means something that takes a lot of effort or skill. **Difficult emotions are feelings that might be challenging for you to think about, manage, or control.**

Everyone has these kinds of experiences. What is important is controlling your reactions and expressing your emotions appropriately to others.

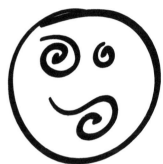

Expressing difficult emotions appropriately or controlling your reactions to them is not always easy, but it's an important social goal. If you ignore difficult feelings completely or "pretend" that they don't exist, you will find it more and more challenging to make them go away. That is, when you ignore difficult emotions, they build up inside of you in a way that can affect you physically (like cause you to feel sick, or make you more likely to get sick) and emotionally (like keep you from interacting with the people that are important to you, or cause you to make decisions that are not appropriate ways to solve problems). So, remember, whatever emotions you have, even the difficult ones, should be acknowledged and dealt with in an appropriate manner.

Below is a list of steps you can take when you are feeling a negative emotion and need to demonstrate self-control:

1. Using what you learned in Chapter 2 about feelings and emotions, decide what you are feeling. Give the feeling an emotion label.

2. Say the label to yourself, either in your head or out loud; it doesn't matter. The simple act of giving the feeling a label will start to move your brain in the right direction to getting calm and moving forward.

3. Get specific and figure out what might be causing you to feel worried, frustrated, angry, or any other difficult emotion.

4. Share your feelings with someone using an "I feel _____ statement." You might choose to talk to an adult that you trust, like a parent, if you are feeling overwhelmed with schoolwork. Or, you might talk with the person who is involved with the situation that is causing you to feel negative emotions, like the friend that you are having a disagreement with.

5. Follow through with a whole conversation. Hearing everything and taking time to think about it will help you deal with the difficult emotions in a more complete way.

If you understand your feelings better, you will be able to deal with them better. Most important, you will be better able to communicate to others what is bothering you and ask for help if you need it.

Suppose you made plans to hang out with a friend on a Friday night. You were really excited to have your friend come to your house to watch a movie and play video games. But at the last minute, your friend had to cancel because he came home from school sick. When you get the message, your first reaction might be to get angry with your friend for canceling your plans. But knowing the difference between "angry" and "disappointed," and recognizing which feeling you are experiencing, allows you to make better choices about how to express your feelings.

In this example, you can't be angry with your friend for being sick. It is reasonable to think that plans will get canceled if someone is sick. It would be more helpful for you to label your feelings about the situation as "disappointment." Feeling disappointment and feeling anger are two different things, and because they are different, most people express them in different ways.

In Chapter 2, you learned how feelings have levels or grades and that you can even measure how "big" a feeling is on a "feeling thermometer." Disappointment is a feeling that is usually less intense than anger. When you are angry, you may make bad decisions or display behaviors that others might consider inappropriate.

In the example above, feeling angry with your friend might make you feel like screaming at him or telling him you never want to see him again – things that would damage a friendship. Feeling disappointment, however, shows that you recognize what's really happening in the situation and that you can move on. **BUT** if this friend is someone who *always* cancels plans with you, and *always* says it's because they are sick, being disappointed so often could make you feel very, very angry. That would make sense since the problem is much bigger. Remember, how you express your feelings when you are dealing with a social problem should match the problem.

Big problems cause bigger feelings that are harder to manage and express. Smaller problems create smaller feelings. You have to match the way you express your feelings to the size of the problem.

On the next few pages, we will talk about feeling calm and provide some thinking and behavior tools you can use to help you with self-control, to prevent losing control, and to "salvage the situation" if you end up having a meltdown.

Staying Calm

Calm is an experience of feeling free from excitement or disturbance. You might be feeling calm when you are quietly watching television or reading a book.

Calm may include:

- Being quiet or relaxed

- Doing things that are quiet or relaxing

- Being "clear-headed": having nothing on your mind but the tasks we have at hand

---

Calm Vocabulary

Synonyms (similar to) – peaceful, quiet, serene, untroubled, restful, tranquil

Antonyms (opposite of) – agitated, bothered, flustered, distressed, tense, worried, on edge, excited

---

How to Calm Down

It is important to try to do something before it becomes too difficult to stay in control of your behavior.

Some things that can be done *before* you lose control include:

- Knowing ahead of time what situations are difficult for you to manage, avoiding those situations, or preparing yourself for them.

- Using the Feeling Thermometer or the Incredible 5-Point Scale to review how you view levels of emotions and how you deal with them.

- Getting help from an adult ahead of time if you know a situation is going to be difficult for you. The adult will probably be able to support you and help you express yourself appropriately.

- Trying one of the calming strategies that are listed on the following page, like deep breathing or talking with someone, will help you maintain focus on your emotions and stay in control.

- If you can, ask a friend (or sibling) who knows you very well to stick by you when they are with you in the situation that is upsetting to you. They can be a model for you, or even help you to recognize when you are losing control and maybe help you change your behavior.

Sometimes you might not be able to demonstrate self-control. You may have a difficult time keeping your body, thoughts, or emotions under control. If your behavior becomes inappropriate for the situation you are in, you will need to make a quick repair of the situation and try to calm down.

Here are some ideas for calming down after you have become upset:

- Take some deep breaths before you say or do anything.

- Do a yoga pose.

- Tense your hands for 5 seconds and then relax your hands for 5 seconds. Repeat this a few times.

- **Stop and Think** about how to change the situation.

- Think about a place that makes you feel calm or happy and picture yourself being there.

- Make up a special cue word that you can use to help you think about calming down when you realize that you might not be using good self-control.

- Move away from situations that make you tense or upset, especially if you have difficulty expressing emotions appropriately.

- Get an adult to help you become calm.

- Find an activity that makes you feel successful.

- Talk it through with another person.

- Listen to music that makes you feel good.

- Exercise! Go for a run, bike ride, a brisk walk, play a sport or get active in some way. Exercise releases special chemicals in your brain that make you feel happy! By the way, exercising on a regular basis can really have a positive affect on your overall mood.

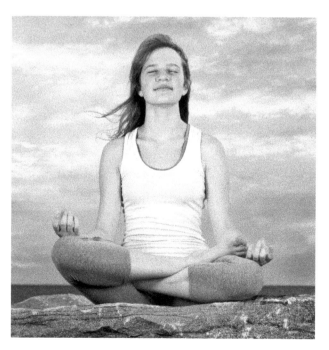

There are a lot of ideas in this list. You need to figure out what will or will not work for you. You can figure this out by trying all of the ideas at different times and seeing how the strategy makes you feel. If it makes you feel more active or "up," it is probably not a good calming strategy for you. If it makes you feel quiet and in control, it will be a strategy you will want to continue using.

"Black-and-White" or "Rainbow" Thinking?

In the introduction to this book, we talked about Big Picture Thinking. You read that Big Picture Thinkers are people who can think "flexibly." They can shift their thoughts from being very specific to being more abstract. To put it a different way, they can change their thinking from being very "narrow" to being much "wider."

Being able to think flexibly allows you to respond more effectively in different situations. For example, you can see all sides in an argument or figure out more than one solution to a problem. You could say that inflexible thinking is **black-and-white thinking** and flexible thinking is **rainbow thinking**.

Black-and-white thinkers have difficulty being flexible in their mind and seeing different possibilities and perspectives. They usually see only one side in an argument or debate, or only one solution to a problem. They are also not very open to trying new things or hearing new ideas. If you are a black-and-white thinker, you tend to see things as either black or white, without noticing anything in between.

Rainbow thinkers are flexible in their minds. They can see many different possibilities and perspectives, and they understand that problems can sometimes have as many solutions as there are colors of the rainbow. They are open to changes, trying new things and hearing new ideas. Rainbow thinkers know that there are more "colors" out there to consider, not just black and white.

Being a black-and-white thinker is good for solving certain kinds of problems because it really helps you zero in on details. Remembering facts and dealing with numerical problems are some of the things that black and white thinkers are good at. But, it's not a great thinking style for social and emotional situations or problems.

Being a rainbow thinker is an important part of being able to see the Big Picture in a situation. Black-and-white thinking focuses more on details and is rigid, which makes it hard to think clearly and flexibly in social and emotional situations. Rainbow thinking allows you to deal with problems more quickly and easily, right in the moment. Social situations, emotions, and communication happen at a very fast rate, and changes are constantly happening that need to be thought about.

Rainbow thinking is a great thinking style for dealing with the rapid changes that happen in social interactions, and it can make you more aware of what to do in social situations.

Self-Talk

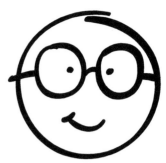

The act of thinking quietly to help you come up with what to say or how to behave, before, during, or after an experience is called self-talk.

Self-talk is an "internal conversation." What you "say" to yourself can help you better understand your emotional state because it usually relates to what you are feeling. It can also create specific emotions inside of you.

Self-talk can be positive or negative, which can change your feeling states to positive or negative. For example, you can feel calm, worried, happy, frustrated, or impatient, depending on what you "tell" yourself. Self-talk can have an effect on your self-esteem, outlook, energy level, motivation, performance, and relationships with others.

Developing a habit of positive self-talk is important. Try to understand your thinking style and label what you are telling yourself. Try your best to change your thought processes for a better outcome. Replace negative thoughts with positive ones. Below is a list of negative thinking styles and how you might want to change them:

- If you tend to focus only on problems, instead, try saying quietly to yourself, "Most problems have solutions. How do I want this situation to be different?"

- If you tend to think that every bad thing is a horrible disaster (complaining), instead, try saying, "Yes, bad things do sometimes happen and that can feel hard, but not every bad thing is a disaster."

- If you tend to expect the worst (for example, by saying, "What if I do terribly on this test?" "The people at that lunch table will never let me sit with them."), instead, ask yourself questions that help you imagine positive outcomes. For example, "What can I do to better prepare myself for this test?" "How can I make a better impression on the people I want to sit with?"

- If you tend to blame others (thinking that others are causing your problems does not help you solve them. It just allows you to avoid being responsible for things), instead, try focusing on what YOU can do to solve the problem. We can't change anyone else's behavior – only our own.

Self-talk can be a great tool for reminding you about social strategies and helping you turn negative feelings into positive ones. It is called self-talk because it is something that you do quietly by yourself. Self-talk is thinking about things in your head; it is not speaking out loud. Speaking out loud to yourself is a behavior that could be distracting to others, or make them feel uncomfortable around you, so remember to use self-talk without making it noticeable to other people.

Go With the Flow

Sometimes you can use key phrases or sayings to help you remember about self-control or expressing your emotions appropriately. "**Go with the flow**" is one of those helpful phrases.

To "go with the flow" is one way of dealing with situations where it is considered important for you to go along with a decision that someone else has made, or be a part of the decision-making process itself.

Think of yourself as a waterfall flowing into a stream. The water keeps moving, always in the same direction. You want to try not to be the big "rock," or tree trunk, that blocks the water from flowing. In other words, people will want you to work with them, not against them. And as long as they are asking you to do something safe, you should try to go with the flow.

You might hear people make comments like these: "Really, Rebecca, everyone else in our group who is working on this project wants to start with making the poster. It would be much easier for everyone if you could just go with the flow."

On the previous page, you read about self-talk. **The saying "Go with the flow" can also be an example of self-talk.** You might use it in a situation where you need to remind yourself to think flexibly. It might sound something like this:

"I know that I usually go to the library to study for tests, but today I was invited to study with Linda. I think I can go with the flow on this, and try a different study method for this exam."

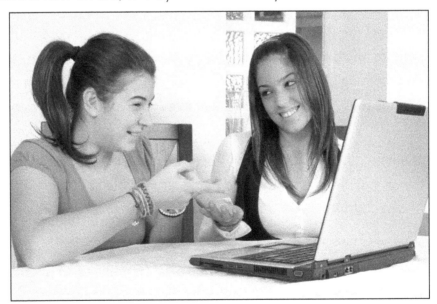

The Incredible 5-Point Scale

The Incredible 5-Point Scale was introduced in Chapter 2. As we saw, it is a tool that can be used to measure emotions. It can also be a good tool to use for self-control.

You can use the numbers 1-5 to represent how your "out-of-control" behavior looks and feels and relate it to a particular situation. You can use the scale before you are in a situation where you know you have difficulty with self-control, and even bring it with you so you can "check in" with yourself while you are there. A slightly different version of the stress scale is found in the Appendix on page A8.

Self-Control

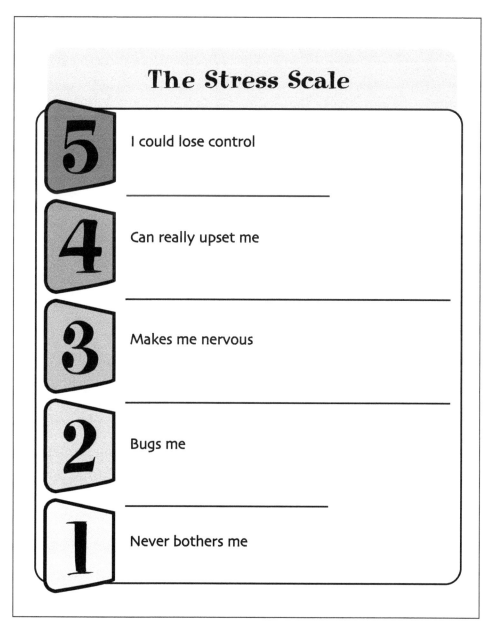

The Stress Scale

5 — I could lose control

_____

4 — Can really upset me

_____

3 — Makes me nervous

_____

2 — Bugs me

_____

1 — Never bothers me

From *The Incredible 5-Point Scale* by Kari Dunn Buron and Mitzi Curtis, 2003, Shawnee Mission, KS: AAPC Publishing. Reprinted with permission.

Ignoring

Ignoring is:

- Not paying attention to something or someone

- Pretending you can't hear something or someone

- Pretending you can't see something or someone

- Pretending someone or something is not there

Ignoring can help you in situations where you might otherwise get into trouble. It can help you stay calm and deal with difficult feelings.

You might need to ignore things like:

- Annoying people

- Distracting noises

- Bothersome brothers and/or sisters

- Teasing

But you don't want to ignore things that are important like:

- Your parents

- Your teachers or other adults when they are trying to talk with you

- Bullying

- When you are not feeling well

Ignoring important adults or a bullying situation can get you into trouble.

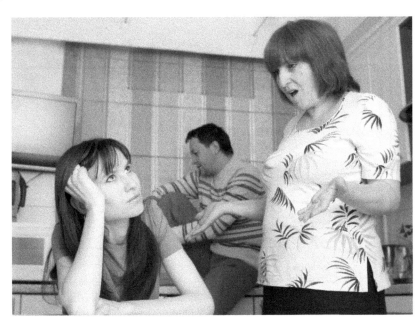

Big Picture Thinking and Self-Control

Showing "self-control" means that you are paying attention to your actions, words, and emotions and that you are able to **Stop and Think** before acting or speaking.

People behave differently in different situations. It is important to make sure you are communicating what you really want to communicate when you are around other people. You also need to try to understand what others consider appropriate behavior when you are with them in school, at home, or anywhere else.

 KIDS IN ACTION REVIEW

The example story at the beginning of the chapter was about Evan, who had a lot of difficulty managing his activity level and staying in control of his behavior at school. Without self-control, Evan's behavior might cause problems for him and the other students in his class.

There are many ways that you can monitor your behavior. Try different things to find out what works best for you. In this chapter, you have read about:

- How the people around you have thoughts about your behavior

- Matching your behavior to the situation around you, remembering that different places have different social rules that you have to follow

- The importance of self-control and strategies that you can use to help you maintain self-control or "salvage the situation," if you have lost self-control in a difficult situation

Demonstrating good self-control is important when you are interacting with others.

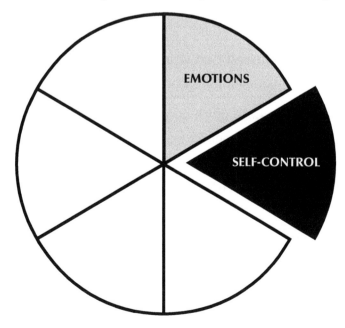

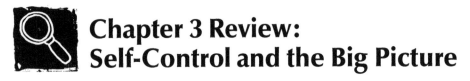

Chapter 3 Review:
Self-Control and the Big Picture

Having control over your behavior and feelings is important when you are interacting with others. People expect different things in different situations, and you need to be able to shift your thinking from one context to the next to behave appropriately. If you understand yourself better, and have better control of your thoughts, words, and actions, you can be more successful socially.

Practice Ideas

1. **Self-Talk.** As defined earlier in this chapter, self-talk is an "internal conversation." Practicing positive self-talk on a continuing basis will help open you up to better ways to solve problems and have better self-control. Your attitude will make all the difference. Ways to practice positive self-talk include:

    -   **Pay attention to your self-talk.** What does it sound like? If it's negative, try to figure out how and why your statements are that way (see page 83). If you are unable to observe yourself and your behaviors, get help from someone who knows you well.

    -   **Reframe.** If you have a negative thought, try to change it, or "re-frame" it, in a positive way. For example, if you are telling yourself, "I'll never get this report done on time," change it to something like, "I'm worried that I won't be able to complete this report on time. What can I do to make sure that I will?"

    -   **Get rid of "absolutes" in your thinking.** Absolutes are words like "always" and "never" that make a situation seem unchangeable. You are capable of doing just about anything, but words like these make it seem like you can't.

    -   **Don't say anything to yourself that you wouldn't say to another person.** Try not to be negative to others; treat yourself the same way.

    -   **Use positive affirmations.** An affirmation is a positive statement that you write down or repeat quietly to yourself on a regular basis to keep your thinking positive. For this to work, you must create a sentence that is in the present tense, positive, personal, and specific. Some examples of positive affirmations include the following:

        -   I am good at _____.

        -   I am always doing the best I can, and so are the people around me.

        -   I am proud that I have great computer skills.

- It makes me feel great to be able to help others.

- I am kind to others and they are kind to me.

Take a look at the examples and decide if any of them work for you. Then, write the numbers 1–5 in your journal or on a piece of paper that you can keep. For each number, create a positive affirmation that you like. Once you have five, you can write, or type in big, bold letters each one on its own sheet of 8½ x 11 paper. Add pictures that go with the words if you wish. Then, hang the pages up in different places where you can see them. Hang one in your room, one on the bathroom mirror, one on the refrigerator, one in your locker at school, anywhere that you will be able to see them on a regular basis. Remember to read them to yourself every time you look at them.

2. **Labels.** When you are feeling overwhelmed by a difficult emotion, take a second to label the feeling. The simple act of recognizing and labeling an emotion can help to organize your mind and calm you. The chapter on emotions (Chapter 2) can help you, and you can practice using the feeling thermometer and the Incredible 5-Point Scale to help you think about how to match the "size" of your emotion to the "size" of a problem.

3. **Use Slogans.** Slogans are a great way to encourage positive self-talk and to help you remember the goals you are trying to achieve. A slogan is a short, catchy phrase used to promote something. You hear slogans all the time in TV commercials so that you will remember the products being shown and later buy them. The section in this chapter entitled "Go With the Flow" is a good example of a slogan that you might use to help you remember to be flexible in social situations. Pick a slogan for yourself. Borrow one from TV or come up with your own. It will help you remember what changes you are working on. Here are some examples:

- "Just Do It" (Nike slogan)

- "I'm Lovin' It" (McDonald's slogan)

- "Be All You Can Be" (U.S. Army slogan)

For example, if you have a hard time enjoying yourself in a certain class at school, you could use the slogan "I'm lovin' it" as an encouraging affirmation statement that you can repeat to yourself privately to help you remember to stay positive. It may feel strange and phony at first, but stick with it. It works!

4. **Practice Calming Strategies.** Find a way, or more than one way, of calming down that works for you. Practice using it when you are not dealing with a difficult moment so you will be prepared when you need it most. If sitting quietly listening to music is helpful, then find 5 minutes a day to do it, whether you need it or not.

5. **Make a List of Helpers.** This would be a list of all of the calming strategies that you have tried and notes about how they helped you or how they didn't help you, and where and when you might be able to use it. Leave space at the end of the list so that you can add more ideas in the future. (You may find a blank copy in the Appendix on page A9.)

Calming Strategy I Tried	Did It Help Me?	When Can I Use It?
Yoga	Yes, I felt very relaxed after.	This strategy is most appropriate for home where I can be alone and relax.
Counting backward from 10 - 1	Yes, it helped me focus on my body and feelings instead of the things around me.	Any time I need to because I can do it in my head.

6. **Make a Playlist.** Listening to music can be a great way to relax. If you like music, it is a wonderful calming strategy. Make a playlist of music that you like to listen to, or music that makes you feel relaxed. Making a playlist is something that you can do on the computer, and an adult, or someone who knows about how to manage music on the computer can help you with that if you need to learn. They will also be able to help you select some appropriate music to include and then show you how to put the music on an mp3 player so you can have it ready when you want it.

7. **Make a "Calming Kit."** It can be something that you keep at home, or something that you can take with you if you need it. Your kit could include things like:

    •   Sensory toys – small ball or stress-reliever toy (fidget)

    •   Pictures of you in a calm or relaxed state.

    •   Music/iPod

    •   A book or something to read

    •   Activities that might help you refocus and take your mind off of other things around you

Developing a calming kit can be something that you can do with an adult, like a parent or a teacher. They can help you brainstorm a list of things that might help you out when you are in a situation where you need to use a calming strategy to help you with self-control.

Chapter 4

The Big Picture: Perspective Taking

In this chapter, we will discuss perspective taking. **Being able to understand another person's point of view about a situation is an important part of communicating and socializing successfully with others.**

Knowing what others are thinking and feeling can help you make better choices about what to say or do. It can also help you make changes in your behavior so that you can keep others thinking about you in a positive way. For example, you need to understand what others are thinking and feeling when you are having a conversation with them. That way, you will know when to join in or initiate a conversation, make changes in the topic, or end a conversation at appropriate times. Understanding what others are thinking and feeling can also help you with knowing what to say and when to say it. These are things that you will have to do in order to get what you need and want from the world around you.

 KIDS IN ACTION: THINKING ABOUT OTHERS

Jimmy and Nadya sit next to each other in math class. Although they are not very close, they have become friendly since the teacher assigned their seats at the beginning of the year. They sometimes work together and talk in class and when they see each other around school.

Today in class, they took a math test that Jimmy had a lot of difficulty with. He finished the test before the period was over and walked up to the teacher to hand in his paper. Nadya watched him walk back to his desk. It was obvious that he was feeling kind of upset. He was walking slowly, with his head down and when he sat down, he sighed very loudly and put his head on the desk. After class, Jimmy looked over at Nadya and said, "That was the hardest test we've ever had. I'm not sure I passed, and now I'm really worried about my grade."

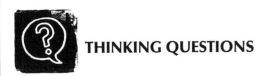

THINKING QUESTIONS

Some nonverbal communication was happening in this story. What is nonverbal communication and what examples do you see here?

Can you pick out the people, place, face-to-face, and word clues that Nadya was observing?

What do you think Nadya said to Jimmy after he told her he was feeling worried?

REWIND

This is a social moment where somebody has given clues about what they are thinking and feeling. First the clues were nonverbal, like the facial expressions and body postures. Then words were used to express feelings. Jimmy didn't specifically say to Nadya that he wanted her to help him feel better, but his words clearly opened up a social moment. Jimmy might have been hoping that by sharing his feelings with Nadya, she would offer him some support and encouragement.

Since Nadya has all the clues she needs about what Jimmy is thinking and feeling, she should know what to say in this situation.

Obviously, you can't see what other people are thinking. You have to use the clues that you **can** see or hear, and what you already know, to help you make guesses about others' thoughts and feelings. Some of the clues you can use include:

- What do you already know about the person you are thinking about?
- What kind of place are you in?
- What's happening right now in the situation?
- What kind of nonverbal cues are we seeing – facial expressions, body language, tone of voice, etc.?
- What are they looking at?

Being aware of the point of view of the people around you is very important. The pages within this chapter will tell more about understanding perspective and how to make smart guesses about what others are thinking and feeling.

Perspective Taking

"Perspective taking" is a term that describes the ability to consider the point of view and motives of yourself and of the other people around you. All the people involved in a social interaction should be keeping track of how their words and personal behaviors affect the feelings of the person or persons they are communicating with. What is important here is that perspective taking is an on-going skill that you need to practice in order to be successful in social situations.

Most people think about each other, whether they are communicating with each other or not.

Imagine (make a picture in your head) that you are on your way home from school with your mom and your little brother. (It's okay if this doesn't sound exactly like your family or what you usually do on the way home from school because it is just an example.) On your way home, your little brother  says he wants to stop at the park. Once you are there, your mom takes your brother over to the swings. You sit down on a bench, which is empty except for your backpack. Your backpack is right next to you. You notice a student from your school who you don't know very well walking toward you. Once you recognize that someone is walking toward you, perspective taking begins – remember people think about each other whenever they are near each other. You might think about why they are in the park and you might be interested to see if they will approach you.

Now imagine that the student you recognized continues to walk toward you. There are many other empty benches around, and since it seems like he hasn't looked directly at you, you "guess" that he is going to sit down on one of the other benches. But instead, without saying anything, he walks right over to where you are sitting. He pushes your backpack to the ground to get it out of the way and sits down on the bench right next to you, so close that your legs are touching. This strange action will probably get you thinking even more about the other person and what he is thinking.

In your head, you might wonder about what is happening. Questions like "Why is he sitting so close to me?" and "Why didn't he just go to an empty bench?" might come up. Or you might be thinking, "This is so uncomfortable." You might also try to decide what to do next, and make a plan to move away or tell the other person to move over.

The thoughts that you have, from the beginning to the end of this situation, are perspective taking in action. You are using the cues around you to help you understand someone else's thoughts and feelings.

Knowing and understanding the perspective-taking process is very important. On the next page you will read about **empathy**, another word that has a lot to do with understanding someone's perspectve.

Empathy

Empathy means trying to understand another person's feelings. It is an important part of social interactions.

Empathy means you are thinking about the thoughts and feelings of others. When you show empathy, or are being empathetic, you are trying to "put yourself in someone else's shoes," to better understand how they are feeling and thinking.

In order to understand how other people are feeling, you must look carefully at their body language and actions. You should also listen to their words and view the situation around you. The People, Place, Face-to-Face, and Word Clues that you read about in Chapter 1 will help you notice more about the feelings of others, and this will help you be more empathetic.

Understanding what other people are feeling will help you do things like:

- Offer encouragement or support

- Know what to say to someone if they are having a problem

- Have a better idea about what to say to someone when you are with them

- Solve problems that might occur when playing or working with others

- Know the right thing to say in a difficult situation

Being a Good Detective: "Social Spying"

A detective is someone who looks for clues and solves mysteries. He makes sure he has ALL the clues before he comes up with a solution. He uses his eyes *and* his ears to do this. Many of the same techniques that detectives use to solve crimes and other mysteries can also be used to figure out social interactions.

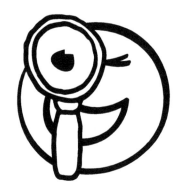

Good social spies look at EVERYTHING – people, places, and things. They know how to look at all the pieces and put them into a whole to understand the Big Picture. A good social spy is definitely a Big Picture Thinker.

Sometimes you might have to act like a detective when you are thinking about the "social world."

Why Be a Social Spy?

A social spy is someone who uses his "detective" or observation skills when interacting with others. Being a "social spy" helps you get information about perspective. It can also help you:

- Solve problems

- Understand other people's feelings

- Find out more about people who you want to be friends with

- Have a better understanding of people you want or need to stay away from, like bullies

- Be a better communicator because you will have the right information about how to start and end conversations, as well as know how to take turns and stay on topic

- Know how to act in certain situations. Picking up on the details around you about where you are and how other people are acting will help you decide how to adjust your behavior if you need to. If you are in a library with your friends, for example, your behavior will be much different than if you were in gym class with them

In Chapter 1, there was a list of clues to look for when thinking about the Big Picture: People Clues, Place Clues, Face-to-Face Clues, and Word Clues. These are the clues that a good social detective needs to pay attention to.

Once you have gotten the individual clues, you can put them together with the information that you have learned from your past experiences to make "educated guesses" about what to do, or about what other people are going to do. They are more than regular guesses; they are "educated" guesses because in making the guessses, you use what you already know about something and then add it to the new information that you have observed.

Making educated guesses is an important part of Big Picture Thinking.

Big Picture Thinking and Thinking About Others

Thinking about others means that you are trying your best to understand the thoughts and feelings of the people around you. Understanding someone else's point of view is also called perspective taking. You have to make guesses about what others are thinking about because you can't see thoughts. You use clues that you can see, along with other information that you have learned in the past, to help you tune in to someone else's point of view.

Understanding the perspective of others can improve your social-communication abilities and your problem-solving skills.

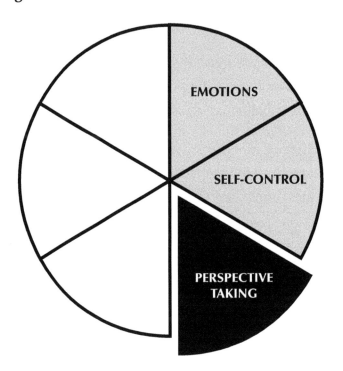

 KIDS IN ACTION REVIEW

Think back to the story about Jimmy and Nadya at the beginning of this chapter. You read about what kind of clues Nadya received from Jimmy, and the Thinking Questions asked you to predict how Nadya might respond. From all of the things that Jimmy said and did, Nadya was probably able to make an "educated guess" about what he wanted and needed at the moment … a little support and encouragement from a friend.

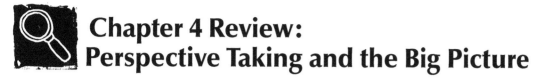

Chapter 4 Review:
Perspective Taking and the Big Picture

You can't be social with others without trying to understand what they are thinking. This is not always easy to do, but you have to try to collect the clues that you can see and make guesses about what people are thinking and feeling in different situations. Understanding the point of view of the people you are interacting with can help you to better communicate, make decisions, and solve problems.

Practice Ideas

1. **Pick a Favorite Character From a Book, TV Show, or Video Game.** Write a letter to that character, thinking about his or her interests and activities. Then, pretend you are that character and write a response to your letter from his or her point of view.

2. **Be a "Social Spy" at School.** Observe what other kids are doing in certain situations like lunch, recess, and gym. You can think that you are a "spy" investigating a case, but keep it in your head. Good spies don't let others know who they are or what they are looking for. That way they are able to get the best clues possible. You can watch from a distance or you can even observe by participating with the others. The idea is just to be super-aware of what is going on around you. After your observation, find time to report your findings in a journal entry or talk about it with an adult that can help you.

3. **Get a Second Opinion.** Getting a second opinion means finding someone else, other than you, to look at or review your work. Once you have done some "social spying," find someone to give you a second opinion about what you have observed to make sure you are on the right track. Picking someone totally different from you might give you a really different idea. For example, choose someone who is much older or much younger than you, repeat Practice Activity 2, and then share your observations.

4. **Learn and Practice the Difference Between "Empathy" and "Sympathy."** Read a dictionary definition of the words empathy and sympathy. These are words that are often mixed up. Think about how they are different and the same. Make a list of situations where you need to be "empathetic" and a list for times you would feel "sympathetic" toward someone you know.

5. **Try to "Walk in Someone Else's Shoes."** Think of a person you could switch lives with for a week. This could be a real or a fictional person. How would it be to do their job, live where they live, hang out with their friends, or do their favorite things. It may not be possible to actually

switch lives, but you might try some smaller activities like eating their favorite lunches for one week or watching a favorite movie of theirs that you have never seen.

6. **Read the Following Common Sayings or Proverbs.** They all have something to do with perspective taking and understanding other people's points of view. Think about what you think they mean and talk about it with an adult. How do these sayings reflect the information that is being talked about in this chapter?"

   - "Actions speak louder than words."

   - "Do unto others as you would have them do unto you."

   - "Great minds think alike."

   - "I felt sorry for myself because I had no shoes – until I met a man who had no feet."

   - "Don't measure your neighbor's honesty by your own."

   - "There are two sides to every story."

7. **Try Perspective Pretending.** In this exercise, you will be changing your own point of view and imagining that you are someone or something else. These exercises can be written like a story or as a list of answers to the questions that are included. You can also talk about them instead of writing.

   - Pretend that you are a "freckle" on someone's face. List some of your "experiences" and some of the comments that you hear going on around you.

   - Pretend that you are an ant at a family picnic. What do you see around you? What do you hear? What are you thinking?

   - Pretend that you are the principal of your school. You have just found out that the president of the United States will be visiting your school and you need to prepare everyone. Think like a principal, and list some of the things you might need to do and some of the people you might need to talk to.

   - Pretend that your family pet (dog, cat, fish, gerbil, newt, etc.) suddenly has learned to talk. What do you think it would say? If you don't have a pet, choose a pet you might like to have and answer the same question.

Chapter 5

The Big Picture: Communication

In this chapter, you will read about communication. **Communication involves exchanging feelings, thoughts, or information.** You can communicate with others verbally (like talking) or nonverbally (like with written words, facial expressions, or body language). In fact, during a conversation, between 50 to 70% of communication is nonverbal – some say the percentage is as high as 93%. We have already talked about some of the elements of communication in earlier chapters, but now we will look at it in more detail.

Communication is an important part of social interactions. You probably have conversations with many different people every day. Sometimes a conversation has a specific purpose, and at other times it is just an enjoyable moment shared with a friend or family member. For example, you might need to have a conversation with a teacher at school in order to ask for help with an assignment that you don't understand. Or, you might be sitting with some friends at lunch talking and sharing fun stories to pass the time. No matter what, you need to remember to think about the "whole" of the conversational moment, not just the parts.

 KIDS IN ACTION: COMMUNICATION

Melissa is a sixth grader, and she's a little shy. She has a small group of friends that she spends time with in school. When she is not in class, you will probably find her with her friends or somewhere quietly reading a book.

Today Melissa is in the cafeteria where she and her friends are eating lunch and talking. Usually she spends a lot of time listening to her friends' discussions at lunch. She often wants to comment or ask questions, and she has a lot of topics that she would like to bring up, especially about the books she reads, but she feels like she never gets a chance. Her friends talk quickly and loudly (it is the lunchroom after all ...), and she has difficulty finding a moment to "break into" the conversation and share her thoughts and ideas.

This can be very frustrating, and Melissa sometimes feels sad and ignored. She talks a lot about this problem at home with her mom. She says things like, "I don't understand why they NEVER let me talk!" or "I don't think they like me very much because they ignore me all the time." Melissa's mom tries to help her understand that she might be seeing things differently than the other girls. After all, when kids are talking, especially when they are in a group, they don't usually wait for everyone to take a turn. Melissa's mom suggests that it might be time for her to change her own communication style if she wants to be included in the lunchtime conversation.

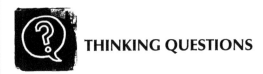 **THINKING QUESTIONS**

What is Melissa's problem?

Do you think Melissa is seeing things differently than her friends?

What conversation skill is Melissa having the most difficulty with?

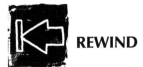 **REWIND**

Melissa's story is an important one. She has a group of friends whom she seems to like, that she wants to hang out with, but she is having difficulty with her conversation skills. Melissa needs to be able to understand how turn-taking works when she is having a conversation with her friends and recognize the right moments to share her thoughts and ideas.

Understanding communication and conversation is important because you need to be able to:

- Be a good listener who shows interest in the people you are talking with
- Share your thoughts, feelings, and ideas with others in a positive way
- Share information with others in a clear and specific manner
- Ask for help from others at times when you need it
- Talk with many different types of people: friends, teachers, parents, strangers, etc.
- Change your style of communicating to fit the audience you are speaking with

Being a good communicator is essential. You need to use good perspective-taking skills and your communication skills at the same time in order to talk with others in an engaging and friendly way. In this chapter, you will read some important things about conversation that will be easy to think about the next time you are speaking with someone.

Communication

Communication is the act of exchanging feelings, thoughts, or information. It happens between people every day in many different ways.

You can communicate verbally (like talking) or you can communicate nonverbally (like with written words, facial expressions, or body language).

This chapter will get you thinking about the following:

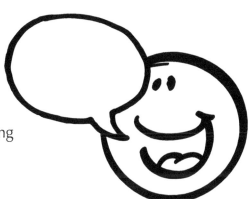

- What is a conversation?

- Why are conversations important?

- What are nonverbal cues?

- How nonverbal cues can give your words more meaning

- Body language

- Personal space

- Eye contact

- Speaking volume

- Tone of voice

- Greetings

- Starting and ending a conversation appropriately

- Choosing a topic, staying on topic, and changing topic when talking with others

- Interrupting, and how certain behaviors can bring a conversation to a close before you are really ready to end

- Joining in a conversation

What Is a Conversation?

A conversation is a common example of how you might communicate with another person. **A conversation is when two or more people talk with each other. They use words to get and give information.**

Having a conversation with someone shows that you are interested in them. And when someone starts a conversation with you, it probably means that they are interested in being friendly with you.

Conversations Are Important

You probably don't give it much thought, but you most likely have conversations with many different people every day, in many different places.

Conversations are an important piece of the Big Picture for you to think about. **Some important reasons to think about conversations include the following:**

- They can help you make and keep friendships.

- They can be a way to ask someone for help.

- They are a way to request information from someone.

- It can make you feel good to talk with other people.

- It can make others feel good when you spend time talking with them.

- They are a way for you to show that you are knowledgeable about something.

- They can help you explain things to other people.

To be good at having a conversation, you must think about what your skills are like and know how to make changes when you are in different situations. You should be aware of where you are, whom you are talking with, and if there is a particular reason you are having a conversation with someone. Thinking about these things will help you communicate with others in a more effective way.

For example, talking with your friends during lunch at school is different than talking with your parents at home during dinner. You will probably choose different topics or words when you are speaking in each situation. It might feel more serious or formal when you are speaking with your parents than when you are speaking with your friends. Similarly, the **volume of your voice** (how loud your voice is) will be different when you are talking with a friend in the library than when you are talking with a friend in the lunchroom at school.

There are different rules about conversation for people of different ages. Younger people engage each other in conversation much differently than older people, and they have different reasons for having a conversation with someone. For example, young children don't usually have lengthy conversations, and the topics they talk about are generally related to the environment, or place, where they are. If they are on the playground, that's what they are talking about. Older people, on the other hand, have longer conversations about a wider variety of topics, and they frequently speak to each other just because they are interested in hearing about the other person and not just because they have a need to get information.

There are also differences between how females and males have conversations. In general, girls of any age are much more interested in talking with others for a long period of time than boys are. And, they generally don't need a specific reason to talk with someone because they seem to like to talk about anything.

And there are different rules of conversation in different countries and even in different parts of the United States. Sometimes where we are in the world has an effect on how we speak to others. This is something for us to think about when we are traveling or meeting people.

Nonverbal Parts of a Conversation

The nonverbal pieces of a conversation can be more important than the words you speak or hear. They add emphasis, or special importance, to the words that are spoken verbally.

When you speak with others, your body also "talks," displaying nonverbal cues to others. When other people speak to you, their bodies also "talk." You give and receive clues about thoughts and feelings from the nonverbal cues the body shows while you are talking with others. **Nonverbal messages are sent to others all the time even when you are just near someone and not specifically having a conversation.**

You might not even be aware of what messages your body is sending, but it is important to try to remember to think about this. It is an important part of getting the Big Picture in a social situation.

Nonverbal cues include:

- Body language
- Personal space
- Volume of voice
- Tone of voice

Nonverbal Cues Add Meaning

Communication is not just about what you say. It's also about what you **DO**. It's about what you do with your face, your body, and your voice while you are talking with others.

The words you speak have meaning, but that meaning can change depending upon:

- How softly or loudly you speak

- How slowly or quickly you speak

- How nicely you say things

- How sincere you are when you say things

- How confidently you say something

- How enthusiastic you are when you say something

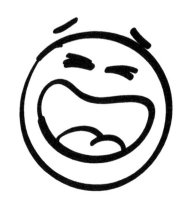

Most people see you as a "whole." Therefore, you have to remember to manage **all** the parts. **Your face, body, and voice give others important clues about what you are thinking and feeling.**

And when you want to know what others are thinking and feeling, remember to focus on the person as a whole first and then decode the parts. **The faces, bodies, and voices of others will give you important clues about what they are thinking and feeling.**

Suppose you are meeting someone for the first time. You might be thinking about saying the right words, but maybe your body language doesn't match what you are saying. Maybe you're telling this person, "I'm really excited to meet you," but you are not showing that emotion with your face because your expression is not smiling and happy. Or maybe your eyes are focused on something else instead of paying attention to the person you are talking with. The person you are meeting will hear your words but also pick up on the body clues that are not matched appropriately. In this case, the person will be receiving a confusing message from you, and that will affect her understanding of what you're feeling and what you are trying to say.

Now, reverse the situation. You are being introduced to someone for the first time. You are focusing on all of the clues that the person's voice, face, and body are "saying" while hearing the words he is speaking. The words say to you, "It's so exciting to meet you," but the expression on the person's face is blank, and instead of looking at you he is paying attention to something else and his tone of voice sounds angry.

If you are able to add up all of the clues you have observed, you will notice that this person's nonverbal cues (voice, face, body) don't match the message their words are sending. As a result, you are receiving a confusing message, which might change your thoughts about what is really going on in the situation.

Nonverbal cues are an important part of being able to understand the Big Picture. Let's now look in more detail at the different kinds of nonverbal cues we commonly use in our culture when communicating with others.

Body Language

It is possible to communicate information to others without words. Some people who are deaf or hearing impaired use sign language to communicate with others. Sign language uses movement of the hands, arms, body, face, and sometimes sounds, to express a speaker's thoughts instead of words.

But all of us, even when we have perfect hearing, use our head, hands, arms, face, and whole body to communicate feelings, thoughts, intentions, and needs – even if we don't mean to and don't pay any special attention to it.

Expressing something with your body is called "**body language**," and this is a big part of nonverbal communication. When you talk with others, your body language adds information to your words, and that gives others more clues about what you are thinking and feeling. You can also receive important clues from the way other people use their body language when they are speaking with you.

Thinking about body language includes monitoring your body postures and gestures and remembering to watch what others are doing with their bodies when you are with them.

Earlier in this chapter, we saw that it is important to match your body language to the meaning of the words you are speaking. That way, you will be sending a clear message to the person you are talking with.

Attending to what other people are doing with their bodies will give you a lot of extra information – this is where being a good "social detective" comes in. People might be using gestures to direct your attention to something or to show you how to do something. Or their eyes and faces might be revealing something about how they are really feeling about the situation.

If you remember from Chapter 4, everyone has thoughts and feelings about the people around them. An important social goal is to understand the thoughts and feelings of the people around you. This is called perspective taking. Body language cues give us a lot of information about what other people might be thinking and feeling.

Personal Space and Proximity: Sharing Space With Others

How close or how far away you are from a person when you are interacting is called personal space or "proximity." **Understanding how people share space when they are together is an important part of nonverbal communication.** Again, it is something we typically don't pay much attention to, yet there are "unwritten rules" for how much space to "use" so as not to send a "wrong" message to others.

You need to think about what your body is "saying" to others. Are you too close or too far when you are talking with them? Standing too close or touching others while you are talking with them can make them feel uncomfortable. Standing too far away will probably make them feel that you are uninterested.

Standing an "arm's length" away when you are talking with someone is the "usual" or common rule.

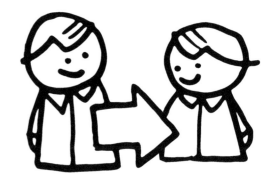

When you are sitting and talking or working in a group with others, you should also think about how close or far away you are. In addition, you should check to see that your body is facing in the direction of the people you are interacting with. This means you are "open" or ready to work or talk with them. When your body posture (sitting or standing, or the direction you are facing) is different from others around you, you will appear "closed" or not available to talk or work with them.

You also have to remember not to touch other people unless they know you are going to do so (like for a hug when it is appropriate; see below). Also, you don't touch other people's things (food, school supplies, personal belongings) without asking. This includes things that might belong to a group of people but are being used by one specific person at a time. For example, if there's only one dictionary in your classroom and someone is using it, it wouldn't be right for you to take it without asking.

You especially need to be aware of personal space when you are meeting someone for the first time. Handshakes or "high fives" are usually the only kind of touching that is appropriate with someone you don't know well. Hugs express that you know a person very well, so you should only be hugging people who are close to you in terms of how well you know each other.

Paying attention to how others share space with you will give you clues about what their thoughts, feelings, and intentions are.

• Take a look at how close or far away they are when they are talking to you or sitting near you

• Observe if they are touching you for a particular reason, like to shake hands or high five, or if they are just so close to you that they are accidentally touching you

• See if they are standing or sitting, or open or closed

• Notice if they ask to touch the things on your desk or if they grab without permission

Sharing space the right way with others will make them feel comfortable when they are around you. When you remember to think about personal space, and how it fits into the Big Picture in a situation, people will feel more comfortable talking or working with you.

Eye Contact

When two or more people are talking, they usually **"make eye contact"** with each other. "**Eye contact**" means that you are looking at the person you are talking with. Eye contact is a "rule" of conversation.

Eye contact is polite and makes other people feel comfortable when you are talking with them. Therefore, it is a part of the "manners" you should be thinking about when you are involved in a conversation.

The secret about eye contact is that you need to use your eyes to get information about what is going on around you. Your eyes help you to pick up on important social cues that are given to you by looking at the bodies and faces of the other people you are talking with.

For partners in a conversation, the eyes and body, as described before, give clues about thoughts, feelings, and intentions. You need to know what these might be so that you can have a successful conversation or interaction with them.

Think of what it is like when you are playing a board game with a friend and the dice roll off the table. Suppose you ask your friend, "Where did the dice go?" and instead of responding with words, she points to the spot on the floor where she saw the dice fall. If you were **not** looking at your friend, you might not have realized that she had responded.

Sometimes it might feel too difficult to look closely at someone while you are talking with them. But you need to give it a try, because it is polite and makes other people more comfortable when they are talking with you. Don't forget that you also need to be gathering information with your eyes to help you better understand your interactions with people.

If you feel very uncomfortable making eye contact, you can try:

- Looking at or focusing on something that is behind the person you are talking with
- Making eye contact intermittently (from time to time)
- Looking at just a part of the other person's face rather than directly into his or her eyes

Voice Volume

Everyone uses their voice to speak. Sometimes you speak loudly and at other times, softly. The loudness of your voice usually changes because you are in different situations or doing different things.

It is important to know whether you are speaking too loudly or too softly when you are talking with others in different places. If you are too loud, it might be uncomfortable for others. If you speak too softly, others may not be able to hear what you are saying.

The "loudness" of your voice is also called volume. Voice volume is a part of thinking about non-verbal communication.

Loud voices are best for when you are on the playground or in the gym at school. You can call this an **outdoor voice**.

As the term suggests, talking voices are best for when you are having a conversation with someone indoors. It can be called an **indoor voice**.

Whispering voices are best for when you are at the library, Movie Theater or some other quiet place, like a place of worship. You might call this a **library voice** to help you remember.

Outdoor Voice	Indoor Voice	Library Voice
Playground	At home	Library
Backyard/outdoors	At a dinner table	Performance: Play or show
Playroom or rec. room at home	In class when it's appropriate to speak	Movie theater
Gym	On the telephone	Place of worship

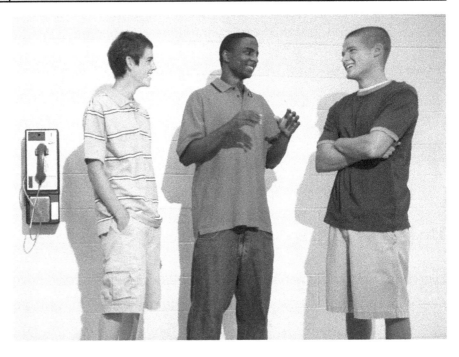

The Incredible 5-Point Scale and Voice Volume

The Incredible 5-Point Scale was introduced in Chapter 2, and another example of this tool was shared in Chapter 3. You can also use the scale to "measure" the loudness of your voice if you are someone who needs to keep track of how loudly or how softly you are talking. You can find a blank copy of the scale in the Appendix on page A10.

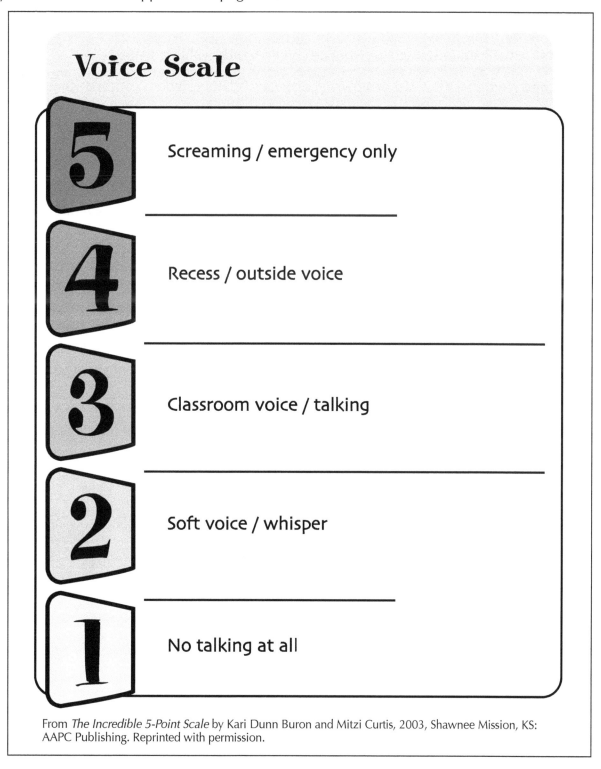

Voice Scale

5 — Screaming / emergency only

4 — Recess / outside voice

3 — Classroom voice / talking

2 — Soft voice / whisper

1 — No talking at all

From *The Incredible 5-Point Scale* by Kari Dunn Buron and Mitzi Curtis, 2003, Shawnee Mission, KS: AAPC Publishing. Reprinted with permission.

Tone of Voice

Tone of voice is a way of describing how your voice sounds to others when you are talking. It's not about **what** you are saying; it's about **how** you are saying it. It includes:

- **Pitch** – How high or low your voice is and how it changes while you are speaking. This is different from volume, because it refers to how deep your voice is. Girls usually have "higher" voices than boys

- **Stress** – How hard or soft you pronounce certain words within a sentence

- **Rate and rhythm** – How fast or slowly you speak and how smooth your speech is

All of these features can change while you are speaking. They might change because you are feeling a certain way, angry or excited, for example; or because you want to express a certain meaning with your words, using humor or sarcasm.

When someone is making a sarcastic comment, you might recognize that their tone of voice is **very** expressive, and there is lots of extra stress or emphasis on each word spoken – as if the speaker really wants you to notice he is speaking completely differently than usual. Easy examples of a sarcastic tone of voice that is meant to be obvious are comments that kids make like "Duh" or "Yeah, Right." Usually, sarcasm is meant to be humorous in the same way as "friendly teasing."

Tone of voice also has a lot to do with your "mood" or feelings. It is hard to have an excited tone of voice when you are tired, or not feeling well. Also, it can be hard to make your voice **sound** sarcastic if you aren't sure about how to do it.

Remember, tone of voice is important. In order to understand the whole message (the Big Picture), it needs to be added in with other nonverbal cues.

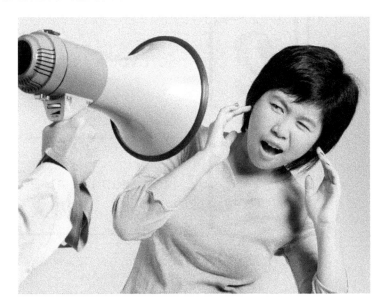

Greetings and Farewells

Greetings and farewells (or "leave-takings," if you need to leave for a moment and plan to return) are a part of our everyday interactions with others. They show others that you are attending to them, and they can help get someone's attention. They are also a "polite routine" (good manners) that you need to remember when talking and interacting with people.

Using a name with a greeting can be helpful. It's a signal to the other person that he needs to pay attention; it can also mean that it's the other person's turn.

Greetings are what you might say to someone when you **start a conversation**. For example, if you want to approach a student in class to ask about working together on a project, you might say something like, "Hi, Emily. I was wondering if you wanted to be my partner for the science experiment."

Greetings can also help you to **join a conversation**. In the example above, you started a conversation with someone who was alone. Suppose Emily was talking with someone else when you wanted speak with her. You could say something like, "Hey, Emily, excuse me for interrupting, but I was wondering if you had a partner for the science experiment?"

Greetings are also used when you **pass someone** in the hallway and want to "just say hi." As mentioned, **using a greeting shows you are polite and interested in connecting with others in a way that you hope will make them feel comfortable.**

Farewells are a way to help you **end a conversation** when you are done talking to someone. Examples include "good-bye," "see ya later," and "I gotta go." Farewells also help you to "**cause a pause**" in the conversation if you need to leave for a moment. For example, "Hang on, I need to go to the bathroom," "I'm going to get that game from the other room, but I'll be right back."

You also might use someone's name with your farewell. For example, if you were finished talking with Emily, the girl in the example on this page, you might end the conversation with something like, "Great talking with you, Emily. I'm excited about working together. See ya later!" This can make somebody feel good about talking with you and help them remember that you are someone that they enjoyed talking with. If there are several people close-by, using a name will also make it clear who you are talking to.

Ending a conversation without a farewell may be uncomfortable and confusing for other people.

More About Social Greetings

Greetings are a part of being social with other people. They are a social routine that everyone expects people to participate in. For example, when you are walking down the hall at school and pass someone that you know, they will probably be thinking that you will make some kind of eye contact with them and say hello, or at least use some sort of greeting gesture, like a wave.

A lot of times, greetings are the beginning of a more in-depth conversation or interaction with others. But at other times, a greeting is just a greeting. That means that the conversation isn't going to go further than a simple "Hello, how are you doing?"

Once you know someone, the next time you see that person, it is important to greet them. As mentioned earlier, people will expect you to greet them. You also need to use a "farewell" as you leave people. There are different ways to greet people in formal and informal situations.

Formal situations are places or events that are "formal" or more serious than others, like an awards banquet. "Formal" can also relate to the person you are talking with, as in someone who you might need to be more respectful to, like the president of the United States or the principal of your school.

"Informal" relates to situations that are probably more common for you, like school or shopping at the mall. It can also relate to the person you are greeting, like someone you know well and see frequently.

Type of Greeting	What Words Might Be Used	Who You Might Be Talking To
Formal Greetings: Arriving	• Good morning/ afternoon/ evening • Hello (name), how are you? **Very Formal:** • Good day, Sir/Ma'am	• Someone you don't know very well • Someone older than you • An authority figure like a teacher, principal • **Very Formal** greetings are for very specific situations where you might be meeting someone VERY important like the president
Informal Greetings: Arriving	• Hi/Hello, How are you? **Very Informal:** • Hey • What's up? • How are you doing? • What's going on? • How's things? • What's happening?	• A friend • Someone you know very well • Someone you see every day

It's important to know that the questions "How are you?" or "What's up?" when used in informal situations don't necessarily need a response. Sometimes a greeting is just a greeting, and no conversation is really meant to follow it. If you do respond, the following phrases are generally expected:

Formal: Very well, thanks. And you?

Informal: Fine/Great!

Unless you know each other well, other people won't expect you to go into great detail about how you are, and if you do, they will probably end up walking away. If someone really wants to know "how" you are, they will be a lot more specific and say something like, "So, I haven't seen you in a while, how are things in school?" Or, they might use your name more directly to indicate that they want to hear more from you, such as "So, I haven't seen you in a while, Joe, how is everything going with your new job?"

Type of Greeting	What Words Might Be Used	Who You Might Be Talking To
Formal Greetings: Leaving	• Good morning/afternoon/ evening. • It was a pleasure seeing you. • It was nice seeing you. • Goodbye. (*Note: After 8 p.m. – Good night.*)	• Someone you don't know well. • An authority figure. • Someone older than you – like an older relative or a friend's parents.
Informal Greetings: Leaving	• Goodbye/bye. • See you (later). • Talk to you later. • See you around. **Very Informal:** • Later.	• Friends, classmates that you see every day. • People that you know well.

Another important thing to remember about farewells and leaving is that people often say things like, "Talk to you later" or "See you later," but that doesn't always mean that you will definitely talk to them later. Sometimes a farewell is just a polite way of ending a brief conversation or interaction.

What makes a lot of this confusing is that there are no clear rules, so if you are not sure, play "social detective" and see/listen to what others are doing and imitate that, as appropriate.

Interrupting

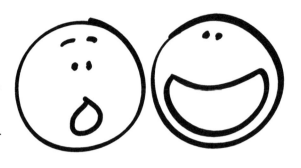

Interrupting is doing something that makes it difficult for people to concentrate. For example, you are at school, and everyone in your class is working quietly on a quiz. Speaking too loudly or making noises could cause a distraction that would make it hard for your classmates to concentrate – it might even make them make mistakes.

Doing something that causes people to stop what they are doing is also an example of interrupting. Suppose you are at home, and your mom is talking on the telephone. This is probably not a good time to ask her a question, but you choose to do it anyway. Maybe you are very careful about how you approach her and how you ask her, but she will still probably have to stop talking on the phone in order to tell you to wait.

Talking at the same time other people are talking also comes under the topic of interrupting. This may be when your teacher is talking to the whole class or when you are having a conversation with another person. Sometimes when people are talking to you, or with you, they might say something that will make you want to comment or ask a question. In such cases, remember to keep your thoughts in your head and wait until it's your turn to talk.

When people are interrupted, they may become frustrated or get angry. They may think the person who is causing the interruption is not fun to be with and may decide to stay away from someone who interrupts a lot.

You might have these feelings too when you are interrupted and can't finish a sentence or complete something that is important for you to finish.

Remember not to interrupt so you don't disturb others when they are thinking or talking.

Conversation: Topics

Conversations are about "giving and taking." Not just taking and not just giving. This means that all the people who are talking get a turn. You need to make sure that you are not doing too much of the talking or not doing enough.

A **topic** is "what" people are talking about in a conversation. Topics usually relate to your interests and everyday experiences, such as movies or television shows, things you did in school, your family, your vacation, your after-school job, etc. In fact, any of your experiences are possible topics for a conversation. The key is to choose from all these possible topics which one to talk about and when to do it.

You need to be aware of topics so that you can keep a conversation going. Keeping a conversation going shows others that you are considering their thoughts and feelings and that you are interested in talking with them.

Choosing a Topic

You have to be a good "social detective" when you are thinking about conversation topics. You can use your observation skills to help you select, change, and continue topics when you are talking with others.

In order to do this, you need to know:

- **Who are you talking with?** Are you talking with an adult or an authority figure (teacher, principal, the parent of a friend?), with a close friend, or with an acquaintance – somebody you know but not very well? Are you talking with a boy or girl who is close to your age, or somebody who is older or younger than you?

- **What is their current mood, or what are they thinking and feeling at this moment?** Are they available to talk with you about what you want to talk about?

- **What is happening around you?** Are you in a classroom or at a sporting event? Are there a lot of other people around the person that you want to speak with?

Choose a topic that is appropriate for the person, time, and place. The next pages will give you examples of how to group topics together to make it easier to understand how to match what you are going to say to person, time, and place.

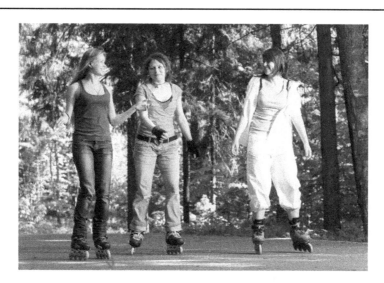

"So I see you like roller skating, too ... do you come to this park often?"

Universal Topics

Universal topics are topics that are easy to talk about with anyone because they are related to life experiences that almost everyone has.

These are subjects that are good to talk about with people you have just met or you are only beginning to get to know, because it is understood that they are "universal" experiences. You don't need to know a lot of specific information about another person, because you can make an educated guess that they have had some experiences that are similar to yours.

Universal topics include things like the following:

Surroundings: This category consists of the weather, the people around you, giving compliments on how someone else or the person you are talking with looks, and other things you can see.

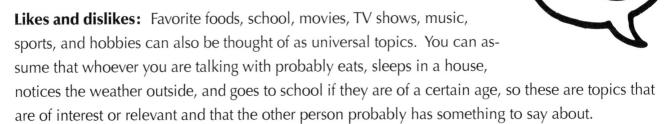

Likes and dislikes: Favorite foods, school, movies, TV shows, music, sports, and hobbies can also be thought of as universal topics. You can assume that whoever you are talking with probably eats, sleeps in a house, notices the weather outside, and goes to school if they are of a certain age, so these are topics that are of interest or relevant and that the other person probably has something to say about.

The latest news: Most people pay attention to the big news stories that are going on around the world, and these can be good examples of more general topics that we can talk about with people we are just getting to know.

Particular Topics

Particular topics are thoughts and ideas that contain more specific information than universal topics. You might need to know a little more about the other person, or ask more questions about them in order to talk about these kinds of things. For example, I like sports, and I can talk about sports with my friend Joe, because I know he's interested in sports, too. But football is his favorite, so he would probably prefer to talk about that rather than my favorite, ice hockey.

Specific television shows, video games, and movies are great examples of "particular" topics. It doesn't mean that you **can't** talk about them. It just means that it might be difficult to talk in depth about your favorites if the person you are speaking with is not familiar with them. For example, I like talking about movies with my cousins Jorian and Melanie because we all like to watch movies. But they love the Twilight series and I haven't seen any of those, nor do I know anything about them. So, if my cousins decide to talk with me about their favorite scenes, they will have to give me a lot of background information so that I can understand what's happening and be included in the conversation.

Personal Topics

Personal topics are topics that are private. If you bring them up, it is possible that you might make the person you are talking with feel uncomfortable.

The general rule is not to bring up personal topics unless you know the person you are talking with very well. You must be pretty sure that he or she will not feel offended by your topic choices.

Personal topics include grades, money, serious family issues, religion, politics, health issues, and personal relationships. There is no guaranteed way to know if what you are going to say will make someone feel uncomfortable. That is why it is important to think **before** you speak.

Understanding the Big Picture and being a good "social detective" will help you recognize if the conversation topic is appropriate for the audience, time, and place. For example, when you are at the dinner table (or any table where you might be eating with others), you wouldn't want to talk about the really violent and bloody movie you saw last night. No one wants to be "grossed out" when they are eating. Although "gross" topics of conversation can be fun at the right time, like when you are discussing a really violent and bloody video game with your friends while you are playing it, you should consider them "off-limits" at mealtimes and with certain groups of people. Think of them as personal topics.

Most personal topics should be shared *only* with your family or the friends who are closest to you and your family.

If you bring up a personal topic, you must be respectful if the person says, "I don't want to talk about it." And if someone brings up a personal topic with you, you have the right to let them know, in a polite way, that you are not interested in talking about it. It is very easy to say something like, "I'm sorry, I'm not comfortable talking about that right now," or "That's kind of personal and I don't really feel like talking about it." The people you are with should understand and move on to something else. If they don't, it is your responsibility to change the subject and move on.

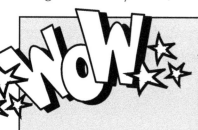

Quick Note: If someone asks you a question that you don't feel comfortable answering, you can respond by asking them something back like, "Why do you want to know?" or "Why are you so interested in knowing about that?" This will make them stop and think about what kind of a question they have asked, and possibly recognize on their own that they may have crossed a privacy line. If not, follow the suggestions above – change the subject and move on.

Starting Conversations With Others

There are different reasons for starting a conversation. There are times when you **want** to start a conversation, and there are also times when you might **need** to start a conversation.

Wanting to talk means that you have something that you want to share with others. You might want to talk when you have a funny story to tell or if something the teacher says reminds you of an experience you have had. Or maybe you just want to have a conversation about something that really interests you. As long as it's a good time for the person or people you want to talk with, you can probably get started.

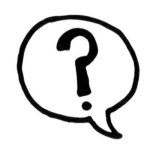

Needing to talk means that you have something important to say that must be communicated to another person in a timely manner. Asking questions in class and going up to a teacher to ask for help are examples of "needing" to talk.

Take a minute to imagine you are in math class and the period is ending. Your teacher has just spent the entire lesson introducing a new concept, but you are not sure that you understand it. It is important for you to let the teacher know that you need help. This would be a time where you **really need** to talk. It is now the end of class, and the teacher and other students are busy packing up and getting ready to go to their next class. There is probably a lot of movement and confusion, and it's possible that other students also want to talk to the teacher. Still, this would be an appropriate time for you to approach your teacher, wait your turn, and politely talk about your need for extra help. You might have to wait for a while before you can interrupt in a polite way. Remember to pay attention to what else is going on around you, because it is the end of the class period, and there is probably only a brief amount of time for you to talk with your teacher.

Now, imagine you are back in math class again. Your teacher is in the middle of teaching the new concept, and you are really enjoying it. Perhaps you have learned the material over the previous summer at math camp and completed a special project using the concept. You **really want** to tell your teacher all about your experiences and what you learned, but the teacher is still talking and all the students are listening quietly. This would be NOT a good time for you to raise your hand and start a long conversation with the teacher about your knowledge of the material. If you do, you will be taking time away from the other students, and the teacher may ask you to stop and continue later on.

Getting Started:

1. **Check to see if it is a good time to talk.** Is it a good time for you and is it a good time for the person you want to speak with? Make sure the person you want to speak with is not too busy to talk to you.

2. **Make sure that the person you want to speak with is not talking with someone else.** If they are, you have to decide about whether you **really need** to talk or whether you just **really want** to talk. If it is important that you talk to the person right away, you may need to interrupt politely.

3. **When you are sure that the time is right, begin the conversation.**

Good Things to Say When Starting a Conversation

Starting a conversation can seem difficult at first. In fact, getting started is probably the hardest part of the conversation. Once it has started, the back-and-forth talking and listening part usually flows much easier.

Again, it is helpful to think about the Big Picture within the situation. What do you know about the person you are talking with, and what is going on around you?

Being aware of these things will help you make good decisions when trying to start a conversation. Don't forget to also think about the other person's perspective, as you learned about in Chapter 4.

Getting Started:

1. **Start with a greeting.** Say something like "Hi" or "How are you?" if you are seeing the person for the first time that day. If you don't know the person's first name, find out early in the conversation (just ask) and use the name within the conversation. You will be considered polite and thoughtful for doing so. As said earlier, using a name also indicates to the other person that it is her turn to talk.

2. **Talk or ask about what the person, or friend, is doing right now.** Look at the situation you are in. For example, maybe you are at a sporting event; if so, you could talk about the game you are watching or suggest going to buy a snack at halftime.

3. **Ask questions about the past.** Ask about the person's weekend, vacation, or holiday, when appropriate. Use "open-ended" questions, which are questions that do not require a yes or no answer but some other kind of answer, because that can help keep the conversation going. For example, instead of asking, "Did you spend the holiday with your family?," which would require a yes or no answer, you might ask something like, "So, Allison, what did you do to celebrate the holiday?" The second question requires a longer response from your conversational partner, and that will help you both keep the conversation going and can be a springboard for new things (topics) to talk about.

4. **Ask or comment on recent happenings in the news**. A lot of people know what's happening in the news, and that makes it easy to start a conversation. Current TV shows that you know the other person watches are also easy to talk about.

5. **Ask about the person's future plans.** Find out what the person is doing after school or over the weekend.

6. **Ask about one of the person's interests.** Find out right away what the person's interests are if you are unsure. You could ask, "So, Lori, what do you like to do in your spare time?" or "What do you like to do when you aren't in school, Lori?" Those are examples of good open-ended question that can get a conversation going.

Don't forget to try to keep the conversation going. **Ask follow-up questions, make comments, and stay on topic.** This means that you don't ask one question and walk away. You also don't want to keep talking only about things that interest you. You have to try to keep the conversation going by thinking about what the other person says and then responding to that. You will hear more about staying on topic on the next couple of pages.

Staying on Topic

Having a good conversation requires that you are both a good talker and a good listener. This means that you are paying attention to when it is your turn to talk **and** when it is time for you to listen. If you can do both, you will have a much better chance of staying on the topic, changing the topic at the appropriate time, and keeping the conversation going.

Staying on topic means that you are **connected** to the conversation and talking about the same idea. Everyone is taking turns talking and listening, and the topic is continued with each turn. When someone else is talking, he or she is the speaker and you are the listener. Usually the speaker asks a question or makes a comment and then provides a pause for the listener to say something. That can let you know it's your turn to speak about the topic. Sometimes the speaker uses your name to let you know it's your turn. She might say something like, "My family is getting a new pet dog. Nicole, do you have a dog at home?" or "You know what I like about your dog Jeter, Nicole?"

What all of this means is that you will have to listen to the words that are being spoken and also use your eyes to help you "listen" to the important nonverbal cues that are being displayed by your conversational partner or partners. For example, if you bring up a topic of interest to you, you must watch the person you are talking with to see if his facial expressions and body language show that he is interested in what you are talking about. If he is looking away from 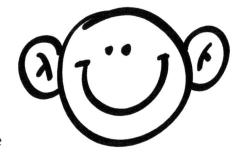 you, looking at his watch or the clock, or showing boredom in some other way with his face or body, it might be time to change the topic or possibly end the conversation.

It is important to stay on topic to show that you are paying attention to the conversation. If you do that, other people will appreciate the effort that you make and will want to talk with you a lot more.

Other Important Things to Remember About Conversation Topics

A conversation requires **cooperation** between speakers in order for it to work well. This means that you and the person(s) you are talking with listen to the words that are spoken and watch for nonverbal information at the same time.

Sometimes topics change quickly; at other times, one topic is talked about for a long time. When you are having a conversation with someone, something that they say may remind you of something **similar**, but not **exactly the same.** This is called a "topic shift," because the ideas are related in some way. Or you might think of something completely different that you want to add. This is called a "topic change," because the ideas are not related.

A **topic shift** might sound something like this:

Jenny: I've been taking gymnastics lessons for three years now, and I'm going to a competition next week. I'm really excited about it, and I hope I win a medal.

Tina: I once won a medal in school for being student of the week.

Jenny: Wow! You won a medal for being student of the week! That's so cool; we only get ribbons at my school for that.

Jenny may have wanted the conversation to continue about gymnastics and her competition. However, her comments about maybe winning a medal made Tina think of the time *she* won a medal. This is a topic shift because the next comment seems to continue the conversation in the new direction.

A **topic change** might sound something like this:

Jenny: I have extra gymnastics practices this week because I have a competition coming up.

Tina: Really? That sounds so exciting. What are you going to be doing there, Jenny?

Jenny: I'm competing in floor exercises and vault. Do you want to come and watch me, Tina?

Tina: Oh, wait a minute. I'm sorry to change the subject, but I just remembered that I wanted to tell you that a few of us are going to the mall after school today. Do you want to come, Jenny?

Jenny: Oh yeah, of course, I will want to do that. But I have to do my homework first, or my mom won't let me go.

Tina: That's fine, we are all going to do our homework at my house, and then my mom is going to drive us to the mall.

Tina wanted to make a topic change and she knew it was going to "interrupt" the topic that Jenny started. She did it in a polite way, and the conversation turned from gymnastics meets to shopping at the mall. They might go back to the original topic, but they could also continue with their plans for the mall. Either way, they are both involved in the same topic.

It's okay if you don't know something about a topic that someone has introduced. Asking questions is a good way to fill in when you aren't completely sure what someone else is speaking about. Use open-ended questions – those not requiring a yes or a no answer.

Talking about the same topic all the time can be boring to others, unless it is something you are both VERY interested in. Think about what you say before you say it and watch the people you are talking with to tell if they are interested.

Changing the topic too much shows you aren't listening carefully or you aren't truly interested in what is being discussed. Moving quickly from one idea to the next can be distracting to the person that you are talking with. She may not be able to help you keep the conversation going.

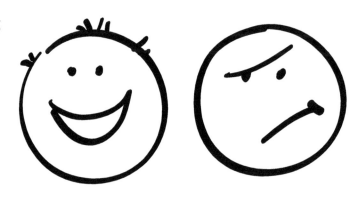

You will know if you are shifting or changing topics too much by watching your conversation partner's face and body for nonverbal cues that show confusion or boredom. Sometimes the person may even tell you that you are moving too quickly, by saying something obvious like, "You need to slow down a little. I can't follow what you are saying."

Also, if someone wants to stop the conversation because they are uncomfortable with the topic, they may say "good-bye," tell you directly that they don't want to talk about it, or simply walk away. Keep an eye out for sudden changes in your conversation partner's words, nonverbal cues, and behavior while you are talking to them. Then you will be able to make a guess about why they may have left the conversation if you are not sure.

Joining a Conversation

Sometimes you might want join a conversation that is already going on. You will need to do this slowly and thoughtfully so that others will be attentive to you and not think you're interrupting or being rude.

1. **Before speaking, observe the people who are talking together.** Even if you can't hear them, you will probably be able to see their gestures (how they move their arms or hands, for example), facial expressions, and body postures. This will help you decide whether you will be able to join in and when.

   People who are involved in a private conversation will be standing close together; you might even see them whispering. Their bodies will be "closed off," which means that there isn't any room for you to stand next to them or near them without moving someone out of the way or tapping someone on the shoulder to get their attention.

2. **Move closer.** After you notice someone, or a group of people, that you would like to talk with, and you have checked to see that their body language and gestures indicate that they are not involved in a private conversation, you can start to move closer so that you can hear what they are saying.

   While you are standing or sitting near them, spend a minute or two listening quietly to the conversation topic and think about whether you have something to share before trying to join in.

3. **Make a brief comment about what is being talked about.** Something like, "I saw that TV show last night, too." Using names helps to indicate turn-taking or a change in turns. If possible, use the name of one of the people involved in the conversation you want to join so that you can get their attention. This is like asking to be included in the conversation. Saying something like, "Oh, Anthony, I totally love that show also, I watch it every week," will give others a good opportunity to respond directly to you.

4. **If you have approached a person or a group and made an on-topic comment, wait and see how they respond.** If the group is going to accept you into the conversation, they will "open up," which means they will literally make room for you to stand with them, look at you, and respond to what you've said to them. If they don't open up, that means that they are not ready to accept someone else into their conversation, and you need to move on to find other people to talk with.

5. **If they do open up, think about what they are talking about.** Even though you may want to talk about your own thoughts or ideas, you are joining a social communication situation that "belongs" to other people. Make comments or ask questions that are on the topic being discussed. Changing the topic right away shows that you are not thinking about others, and it could frustrate and upset them.

Having a Great Conversation

Good conversation skills are an important part of socializing with others. They can help you meet new people or get to know someone better, and they give others an opportunity to get to know you.

Here are some ideas for having a great conversation:

- **Be interesting.** You probably have a large amount of knowledge that you can take ideas and topics from. Make sure that you use it. Picking the same topic over and over again generally bores other people.

- **Show interest.** The people you are talking with should think that they, and the conversation that you are having with them, are important to you. Show interest in the topics that they introduce by asking questions and making comments. You can also try to introduce topics that you think will interest them.

- **Remember to take turns.** This is very important. Your job in the conversation is to talk **and** listen. You should be sharing the conversation equally with your partner. You can sort of measure this by remembering that, in general, if two people are talking with each other, they will each 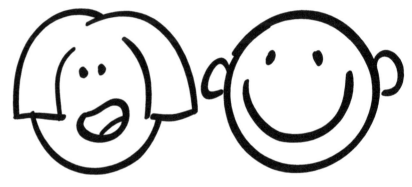 be talking 50% of the time and listening the other 50%. If the conversation includes three people, the percentage would be approximately 33%, and so on.

- **Don't interrupt.** Wait until the person has finished talking before you comment or ask a question.

- **Be focused.** Try to stay focused on the person you are speaking to. Make eye contact and pay attention. Using good manners such as these makes others feel more comfortable around you.

- **Use your eyes, not just your ears, to listen.** Remember that your eyes help you see any nonverbal cues that are being displayed by the person you are speaking with. You need to put the visual information with the verbal information that you have taken in so that you can navigate, or find your way through, the conversation better.

- **Keep it going.** Answer questions completely. Always try to think about something else you can say but make sure it is related.

"Conversation Crushers"

"Conversation crushers" are things that happen during a conversation that cause it to come to an unexpected end.

Examples of conversation crushers include the following:

- **Interrupting.** This could be talking out of turn or displaying behaviors that are distracting to your talking partner, like looking away, making noises, moving your body instead of standing still, or walking away.

- **Not thinking about the topic.** These are things like changing the topic too much, not staying on the topic, or staying on a topic for too long. If you change the topic too much, you make it difficult for the person you are talking with to follow along with what you are saying. If you talk for too long about a topic that the person you are speaking with doesn't know a lot about and is not interested in hearing about, he will probably figure out some way to stop talking with you.

- **Not being specific.** When you talk with others about your experiences, it is important that you give them **enough information** so they can understand what you are talking about. For example, you wouldn't tell your friend about a trip to the mall by saying something like, "I went to that place that has all those things … and I bought some stuff." How will she ever know what you are trying to tell her?

- **Being too specific.** Sometimes you might give **too much** information when talking about your experiences. Instead of providing a quick summary, or giving the main idea about an experience, you might give more information than you need to, and, as a result, your listener might get bored and want to walk away.

  Using the example from before, suppose your friend knew you were going to the mall and asked you about it. Maybe you responded by saying something like, "First I got in the car with my mom and my dad and my sister and my dog. My dad was driving, my mom was sitting in the passenger seat, and my sister and I and our dog were in the backseat …" That's a lot of things to say, but not much of it actually answers your friend's question. Continuing in that way will surely be **too** much information.

- **Talking *TOO* much.** Conversation is about giving and taking equally. Not giving someone else a turn, talking too much, or not talking enough when it is your turn makes a conversation very difficult.

- **Not thinking about what your conversational partner needs or wants to hear.** Talking only about what interests *you* shows your listeners that you are not thinking about them. You are only thinking about you. Also, if you forget to watch for nonverbal cues from your listeners to see if, and how well, they are following along is also a way to bring a possibly good conversation to a very quick close.

- **Not keeping the conversation going.** Giving one-word answers to questions or not following a yes or a no with an appropriate comment, question, or example can stall a conversation. No one likes a conversation where they are doing all the giving.

Remembering these things, and working at NOT doing them, will help you have more successful conversations with others.

Big Picture Thinking and Communication

Having good communication skills is an important part of successful social interactions. You need to use good perspective-taking skills while you are communicating with others so that you can have better conversations.

Conversations happen between different people in many different situations. You have to adjust your conversation style to fit the person you are speaking with and the context you are in. **Thinking flexibly is very important if you are going to be a good communicator.**

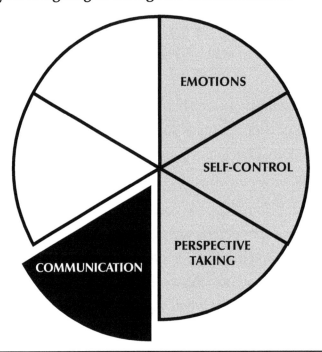

 KIDS IN ACTION REVIEW

The example story at the beginning of this chapter got us thinking about Melissa and the difficulty she was experiencing with her conversation skills. It is very possible that Melissa wasn't picking up on all the clues around her, and that's what was making it so hard for her to talk with her friends at lunchtime.

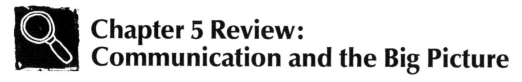

Chapter 5 Review:
Communication and the Big Picture

Communication is sharing thoughts and ideas with others both verbally and nonverbally. When you are talking, the words you use are important, but the way you organize and speak those words can give them even more meaning to a listener.

Conversation is an important part of socializing. Other people will want you to participate in conversations, and they will expect that you are going to follow the rules of conversation.

Practice Ideas

Nonverbal Communication Ideas:

1. **"Mirror, Mirror ..."** As you did in Chapter 2, practice the facial expressions that match certain feelings. Then perform your "faces" for someone and let the person guess which emotion you are displaying.

2. **"Something in the Room."** This is a fun game to play with a partner. A parent, teacher, or friend might be an appropriate choice for a partner. The actor tells the person who is guessing (the "guesser"), "Something in the room is making me feel _____." (Fill in with any emotion like sad, frustrated, or confused.) The actor then directs his eyes toward an object in the room and makes a facial expression that matches the emotion he mentioned. The "guesser" must follow the actor's eye gaze to select the correct object.

   Make this game a little easier by putting objects of different shapes and sizes on a large table in front of the players. That way there is less distance to view between the "eyes" and the object. Make it even easier by taking out the facial expressions and emotions. The actor can just "look" at something in the room and the guesser can simply figure out where the actor is looking.

3. **Tone of Voice Charades 1**. Make two sets of index cards: one pile with emotion words and one with short sentences or sayings of any kind. The object of the game is to match the emotion to the sentences so that they are related. For example, you might write the word "confused" with the sentence "I don't understand this math assignment." You should have more than one "sentence" card for each emotion. Choose a card and try reading the sentence with a "confused" tone of voice. Don't tell your audience what emotion you are performing and see if they can guess. As you improve, try performing the emotion without letting them see your face or body. Can they guess the emotion only from your voice?

4. **Tone of Voice Charades 2**. Make two sets of index cards: one pile with emotion words and one with short sentences or sayings of any kind. Mix up the cards. The actor chooses one card from the emotion pile and one card from the sentence pile and then performs the sentence using the tone of voice appropriate for the emotion listed on the card. In this version of the game, you might choose the emotion word "confused" and then a sentence card that says, "Let's get this party started!" Obviously, the emotion and the words don't match, but you will still need to make it sound like you are experiencing that emotion.

5. **Mute.** Turn off the volume on a TV show or movie. Watch with another person and see if you can interpret the characters' emotions. How much of the show can you understand without listening to the sound?

6. **Gesture and Posture Charades.** With a partner, perform as many gestures and postures as you can think of. Guess the meaning behind what each person is performing. Some ideas could be: Stop! Come here, bored, thinking, and cheering.

Conversation Ideas:

1. **Conversational Practice.** Make a topic box out of a shoebox or similar container. Write possible topics of conversation on index cards and put them in the box. Suggestions for topics include things like:

   - **School** – gym class, a big test, your favorite teacher, what you like to do at recess/or during free time

   - **Home** – siblings, your room, your mom's cooking, things you like to do at home

   - **After-school activities** – sports, place of worship, Scouts, computer games

   - **Friends** – best friends, things you like to do with friends, parties

   Choose an index card and talk about the topic for about 1 minute. (You can set a timer to help you know when 1 minute is over.) Try the same exercise using a timer set for 1 minute and 15 seconds. The goal of this exercise is to try to increase the length of time you can carry on a conversation on a given topic, so keep track of the time; each time you begin, add 15 seconds on to the total time.

2. **Changing the Topic.** This is a variation of exercise 1 above. Before you choose a topic and get started talking, designate a person to be the "topic changer." The "topic changer" chooses a second topic without showing it to you and holds on to it for later. The exercise starts the same way as described above. You choose a topic and talk about it for about 3 minutes, only this time, don't use a timer. It is the "topic-changer's" job to try to make an appropriate topic shift so that the conversation can continue on to the next topic.

3. **Personal Topics.** Make a list of as many personal topics as you can think of so that you can be prepared for future conversations. Remember that some topics are only appropriate for talking about with someone in your family. Do not bring these topics up with certain people or at certain times. Remember that you don't have to respond to others if they introduce these types of topics. What might you say to someone who is talking with you about something that you feel is private?

4. **Conversation Rules.** Go back through the chapter and make a list of all the conversation "rules" that you read about and add any others you can think of. Have two different conversations: one where you follow all the rules and one where you don't. Which one was easier? Which one was harder? Are there any rules that you forgot to put on the list? You can ask an adult to help check your list or add to it.

5. **Questions Only.** Have a conversation with a partner without making any statements – only ask questions! It sounds kind of strange, but it will force you to think about how you are speaking and what you are saying to your partner.

6. **Only "You."** Have a conversation with a partner without making any statements about yourself. Your partner can talk about an experience that she had and you can practice listening. Keep the conversation going by making statements and asking questions about her experience, not by sharing your experiences. Don't use words like "I," "me," and "mine" because when you use these words you are probably talking more about yourself than about your conversational partner.

7. **Big Picture Context Role-Play:** Perform conversation role-plays based on Place, Person, Purpose, and Topic. Look at the suggestions in the lists below to get started.

Find an adult or another person to be your partner. Each time you start a role-play, remember to think about how you will consider each of the categories. For example, the first two role-plays are located at the "library," but the audience, topic, and purpose are different. Although there may be some things about these two role-play conversations that are the same because they both take place in a library, there will also be things that are different. For example, you may be using a "library" or quiet voice volume for both, but the way you talk with a librarian will be different from the way you will speak to your friend.

Location	Person	Purpose	Topic
Library	Librarian	Asking for help	"I think I need some help finding a book for my book report."
Library	Friend	Sharing information	"What you heard is going to be on an upcoming test."
Classroom	Teacher	Sharing an opinion	"What do you think about having school on Saturdays?"
Classroom	Study partner	Sharing an opinion	"I think that you might be wrong."
Video game store	Store clerk	Requesting information	"When is the new version of this game coming out?"
Video game store	Friend	Sharing an opinion	"Which video game system do you think is better?"
Lunchroom	Friend	Sharing a secret	"I failed the math test last week."
Lunchroom	Lunch aide/ teacher	Reporting information	"Someone at another table just threw food at me."

Once you have gone through these suggestions, see page A11 in the Appendix for a blank copy of the chart. Fill in the chart for your next role-play game.

Chapter 6
The Big Picture: Relationships

In this chapter, you will read about relationships. Relationships are connections between people. You have relationships with family and friends. You also have relationships with many other people that you see on a regular basis, like teachers, members of a club you belong to, people in your neighborhood, or people at work when you have a job.

The people in a relationship usually have an effect on each other. They share their thoughts and feelings and do activities together. They are "dependent" on each other, and because of this, when things change for one person in the relationship, it usually has some level of impact on the other person(s) involved. No matter what your feelings are about the people in your life, you have a relationship with every one of them.

When building and maintaining relationships with people, you need to be able to:

- Know which people you are closest with

- Understand the different types of relationships and friendships that you have with others

- Know where to go to meet people and how to form friendships with the people you meet

- Know how to introduce yourself as a first step in getting to know people

- Decide whether a person you meet is someone you would like to be friends with

- Remember the things that you learn about your friends

- Maintain your friendships

- Understand how your behavior can affect your friendships – both positively and negatively

- Recognize when someone else is not being a good friend to you

KIDS IN ACTION: RELATIONSHIPS

Angela and her family have just moved to a new town. She will be starting in the sixth grade at a new school where she doesn't know anyone, and this is making her feel very nervous. Angela tells her mother that she is worried that she is not going to make any friends. Her mother reminds her to use her good "social detective skills" and to spend time observing the other students because that will help her better understand their thoughts, feelings, and interests. Mom also tells Angela that she should think about how she communicates nonverbally with the other students. She tells Angela, "Remember to use some **body language**. Smile and try to sit close to some of the kids that you think you might be interested in meeting. That will help them understand that you are trying to get to know them."

On her first day, Angela walks into her new homeroom class, and her teacher introduces her to everyone. During the introduction, Angela stands at the front of the room. She remembers what her mom told her, tries to stay in control of her anxiety, and puts a big smile on her face. Later, she is happy that she did remember her mother's advice because it worked! Two girls approached her after class and introduced themselves. They let Angela know that they were interested in getting to know her better by asking her to sit with them at lunchtime. Angela and her two new friends, Samantha and Michele, sat together in the cafeteria and took some time to talk to each other about their interests. Angela was really happy to know that both girls loved gymnastics and singing, just like her. She also learned that they were in the school chorus, which made her even happier since she also liked singing and wanted to pick chorus as one of her elective classes.

When Angela went to her next class, she felt more confident about meeting new people and decided to try saying "hi" to a girl who looked at her and smiled. Angela took the seat next to the girl. The two of them introduced themselves, and when class was over, they shared their schedules and Angela found that this girl, named Susan, was in her next class which was science. They decided to walk to class together and were able to talk with each other on the way.

At dismissal time, Angela saw her three new friends again. She made sure to say "good-bye" and "see you soon" so that they would remember her the next day. On the bus ride home, Angela thought about her day. She was very excited to tell her mom all about the new girls she met. Making friends wasn't so hard after all!

 THINKING QUESTIONS

How was Angela feeling before her first day at her new school?

How do you think Angela felt at the end of her first day at her new school?

What do you think Angela told her mother when she got home?

How do you think Angela's second day at her new school went?

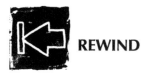 **REWIND**

Making friends and talking with people that you don't know well can make you feel nervous and worried. Angela was lucky to have her mom to help her organize her thoughts and plan what to do before she left for school. There are a lot of details to remember and clues to pick up on before being able to get close to others. But as we saw, it can work!

Having relationships with others, trying to be a good friend, and having good friends also requires good communication skills and good perspective-taking skills, so don't forget the work you have already done in previous chapters. The pages in this chapter will explain some important things about friendship that will be helpful the next time you are thinking about making new friends or communicating with the friends that you already have.

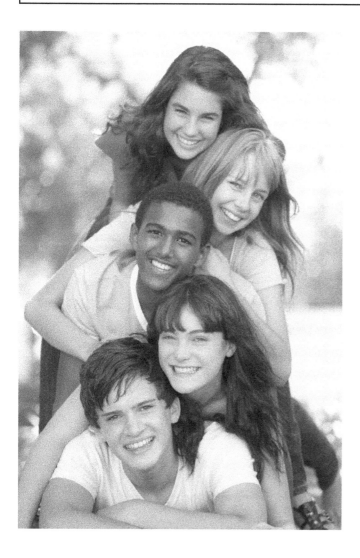

Relationship Building: How Close Are You?

You probably have several people in your life that you call "friends." A friend is someone you have gotten to know, who you like to talk to and spend time with. **You might have more than one friend, or you might have different groups of friends.** For example, you might have friends that you see mostly at school or friends that you know from your neighborhood.

Relationships develop into different levels of closeness, depending on the people, how they meet, how much they see each other, how long they have known each other, and what level of closeness they feel comfortable with. You can think about levels of relationships like steps that show how close the people you know actually are to you. Think of yourself at the top. The steps that are closest to you show closer, more important relationships.

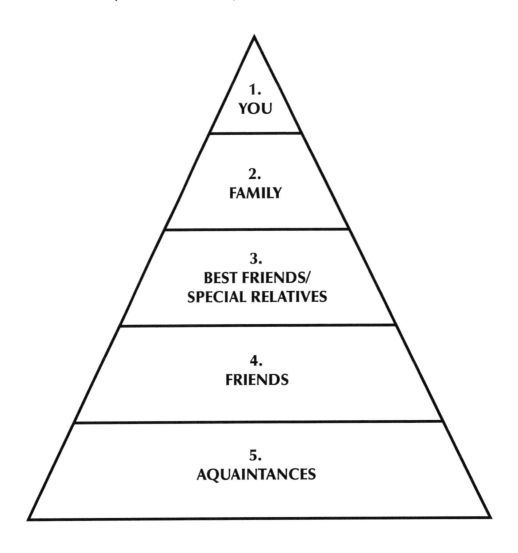

Step 1 is **YOU** on the top step. It represents the relationship you have with yourself.

Step 2 indicates the people that you are closest with. Closeness can be both physical and emotional. This step is usually family members, like your mother, father, and siblings. It can also include a special person like a boyfriend or a girlfriend, if you have one.

Step 3 is for other people, besides your family, that you feel close to. This can be a best friend (or more than one best friend), or other adults that you feel physically or emotionally close to, like an aunt or uncle. Grandparents or other relatives might also be here on this step, or above on level 2, depending on how close you feel to them.

Step 4 is for friends. These are friends that you know and see a lot, but maybe you aren't as close with them, physically or emotionally. These are people who you probably see on a regular basis, like in school or at your favorite after school classes, sports teams, or other activities. You probably feel comfortable talking and hanging out with them when you see them, but maybe you don't see them frequently or feel as close to them as you do other people.

Step 5 is for acquaintances. An **acquaintance** is someone you might know from school, or church, or a club or activity. Maybe you see that person on a regular basis, but you don't spend much quality time doing things or talking with them. "Quality time" is a way of saying that you are spending time with a person, away from the place you see them every day, doing things you like to do together.

It is very likely that some people who are in your life may change steps. For example, you may know someone at school who you consider to be an acquaintance (5). Suppose that you become closer with that person and start sharing more things with them. Maybe you begin seeing them more frequently outside of school. In this example, that person may move from being just an acquaintance, to being a friend (4). On the other hand, maybe your best friend (3) from elementary school moves on and goes to a different middle school. You don't see each other as much and you don't stay close because of that. They might move from being your best friend (3), to just a friend (4), because you aren't spending as much time with them.

Groups of Friends: Building Closer Relationships

You just read about "levels" of closeness that you might feel with the people in your life. Now think a little more about the people you consider your friends or best friends.

You might have different groups of friends that you know from different places. But within those groups, you might notice that you tend to hang out with or talk to the same few people. These people may become closer to you and form a bond with you. You might say that they become your "inner circle" – a group within a group.

Your "inner circle" of friends usually includes people who have the same interests and the same likes and dislikes as you do. They also probably have similar abilities and compatible personalities. For example, you may have a group of friends that you know from a sports team that you play on or dance class you take. Or, you might have a group of friends that you know from Boy Scouts or Girl Scouts. Or maybe you have a group of friends that you hang out with because you've been in the same class since preschool. Getting to know people in these different ways or knowing them for longer periods of time can lead to closer friendships.

There are some differences in the way girls and boys behave when it comes to friends. For example, girls talk to each other a lot more than boys on the phone and in person, and boys tend to do more physical activities together than girls do. But, The Big Picture about "inner circles" of friends is pretty much the same. Your friends are a lot like you, but they also appreciate your differences.

"Inner circles" of friends begin to develop in elementary school. They usually start off small, like two or three friends, and in middle school, they might grow to include more friends. In elementary school and middle school, if you are a girl, your closest friends are probably girls. If you are a boy, your "inner circle" is probably made up of boys. This stays the same until you get to high school. Then boys become friendlier with girls and start to include them in their "inner circles," and girls start to include boys in their "inner circles."

Relationships change as you get older. You may grow closer to some friends and further apart from others. This is a typical pattern.

It has a lot to do with the fact that you change schools, interests, and activities as you get older and so do all of the people you have relationships with. Even so, you may have friends that you have known for a very long time who will always be there for you.

What kind of people should be friends?

- Someone you can trust who knows that he or she can also trust you.
- Someone who likes you and wants to spend time with you.
- Someone who is generous and is willing to share thoughts, feelings, and other things with you.
- Someone who is kind to you, treats you with respect, and acts that way on a regular basis – not just when they want something from you or to show off in front of others.
- Someone who has some of the same interests as you and enjoys doing things with you even when it's not their favorite thing.
- Someone who is willing to help you when you ask for it or notices that you need help and offers it.
- Someone who encourages you when you need support.
- Someone who is easy to play or hang out with.

If you want to, you could keep adding to this list. There are many qualities that make someone a good friend.

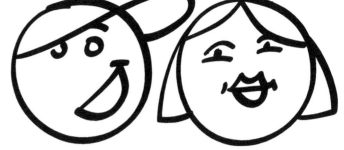

Making friends and keeping friends are important social goals for everyone. Just knowing someone from school or some other place, somebody you don't even interact with much when you do see them, doesn't automatically make them a friend.

What we are describing here are the people that you have close, meaningful relationships with.

Best Friends

A "best friend" is someone who has all of the qualities of being a "friend," but the relationship you have with them feels even closer. Your best friends are usually people who you have known and been friends with for a long time. **It's not typical that kids make a new friend and instantly become best friends** because the closeness in relationships takes time to develop and grow.

Younger children might call all of their friends best friends because they don't have enough "friendship experience" to know the difference. Girls usually talk about having a best friend more than boys, but that can change as they get older. Up until high school, girls mostly have best friends who are girls, and boys mostly have best friends who are boys. After that, boys may have best friends who are girls and the other way around.

If you have a best friend, or more than one best friend, you might notice some of these things about them:

- They are usually close friends whom you have known for a long time, or that you have spent enough time with to get to know them very well.

- They are friends that you enjoy spending a lot of time with. Maybe you spend most of your leisure time with them.

- They are people whom you trust completely. This means that you can share secrets or personal information with them, and they will respect your trust. That is, they will keep secrets if you ask them to, etc.

- They are someone that you are so close with that it is not hard to forgive them if you have a small argument or a disagreement.

- Their behavior toward you stays the same. This means that they **always** display the qualities that make them your best friend. For example, someone who is trustworthy enough to be your best friend should **always** be trustworthy.

- Their feelings about you and your friendship are the same as yours. This means that if you think of someone as a "best friend" they also think of you as a best friend.

Earlier, we discussed "inner circles" of friends. The whole idea of an "inner circle" is that you have more than one close friend around you. And that circle can always be open for more. You can also have more than one best friend or have close friends from different groups.

Your friends also have friends, and possibly they have more than one best friend. Rather than letting this bother you, or making you envious, look at it as an opportunity to meet and get to know other people and make new friendships.

Making New Friends

Making new friends can seem hard, but being aware of and trying some of the ideas here will make it easier. Every day, you are in places where there are other people around. School, your neighborhood, sports events, and the park are all good places to meet people who you could possibly become friends with. To make the best of these opportunities, remember the following:

Put yourself in places where you will find others with similar interests. It's a fact that most people have friends who like the same things as they do. If you want to make new friends, think about your interests and go to places where there will be others who are interested in the same things. Here are some examples:

- If you love playing chess, join the Chess Club at school.
- If you love to play soccer, join a soccer league in your town.
- If you love animals, volunteer at a local animal shelter.
- If you love reading, join a book club or form your own.
- If you are good at a particular subject in school, let the teacher know that you would be interested in helping other students who could use some help with that subject.

Be available to others when you are around them. This means that you make yourself "open" to connecting with others. Ways to do this include:

- **Smiling** – Remember that your body language and facial expressions (see Chapter 5) are what people will see first … before you ever even say a word.
- **Talking** – Remember your good conversation skills (see Chapter 5). Show interest in others who are showing an interest in you. Strike up a conversation with someone and recognize when someone is trying to start talking with you.

- **"Unplugging"** – You won't notice if someone is interested in connecting with you if you are always plugged into some type of technology. Things like playing with your phone and/or talking on it, checking your email, texting, surfing the web and playing handheld computer games make others think you are "too busy to talk" or happy being alone. Listening to your mp3 player with headphones or using any other technology all the time will make you seem unavailable and unapproachable to other kids, not to mention that you will be completely tuned out to what's going on around you. So "unplug."

Use your "social spying" skills. Be a good observer. Look around the room and watch other kids. Pay attention to their nonverbal communication. Look for smiles and gestures that show that they are open to starting a conversation.

Making Introductions When Meeting People

Introductions are a good way to get to know someone when you first meet them. It's important to try to learn someone's name when you meet them, and you should want them to learn your name if you've never met them before. It's okay if you forget a name later. You can always ask the person to tell you his name again.

Sometimes you will need to introduce yourself to other people, and at other times you will need to introduce other people to each other.

Introductions are a good way to begin a conversation with someone you don't know.

Introducing yourself is friendly and polite, and it makes a good first impression. Making a good first impression and appearing friendly lets others know that you are "interested and interesting." Reviewing the skills in Chapter 4 on perspective taking and in Chapter 5 on communication will help you with making introductions, and the suggestions on the following page will give you some specific ideas about how to make introductions.

Introducing Yourself and Others

Introducing yourself:

- Look at the person you are speaking with.

- Use a pleasant voice: Speak clearly and loud enough to be heard.

- Offer a greeting. Say something like, "Hi, my name is, Robin. What's yours?"

- When you leave, say something like, "It was nice to meet you, Robin."

- Always try to remember to introduce yourself when meeting someone new.

Introducing others:

- Stand or sit near the person or people you are introducing to each other.

- Use a clear voice.

- Say the person's first name so that the people around you can hear.

- Give some more information if you think it is important. For example, say where you know each other from, how long you have known each other or even maybe a common interest.

So, let's say you wanted to introduce Bruce, a friend who lives next door to you, to your cousin Danny, who is visiting from another state. You see Bruce in his backyard, and you and your cousin walk over to him. You would probably want to say something like, "Hey, Bruce; this is my cousin Danny from Detroit. He's in the same grade as us, and he is really good at playing *Star Wars Battlefront II* on X-box. You want to hang out and see if we can beat him?"

Remembering Facts About Friends

When you make new friends, you get to know more about them as time goes on. You learn things about them from talking to them and observing them closely (their clothes, hairstyle, games and activities they like to play, etc.).

It is important to get to know things about your friends. It makes other people feel good to know that you are thinking about and showing an interest in them. Also, knowing something about them helps you know what to talk about with them. In Chapter 5 about communication, we talked a lot about topics and starting conversation. The things you know and remember about your friends make good topic choices for conversation.

Store what you learn in your head so that you can find it when you need it. For example, you might let a friend know that she is important to you by remembering that her birthday is coming up or by remembering that she just got a new puppy and asking questions about it.

You might need to remember facts about your friends when you need to start or continue a conversation, suggest an activity that both you and your friend will enjoy, or buy a gift for a special occasion.

Making Friends: Friendly Behaviors

Making friends takes work. You will need to use good perspective-taking skills, because understanding how others are thinking and feeling about you and the situation you are both in is important when dealing with friends. You can review Chapter 4 if you need a reminder about perspective taking.

The following is a list of "friendly behaviors" that can help you make a good first impression when meeting new people. They can also help you maintain your friendships. The Big Picture here is that they are also behaviors that everyone should demonstrate. Remembering to think about these behaviors when you are talking or working with anyone, whether they are your friend or not, is a good thing.

- **Be caring.** Listen and think about what others say. Help others when they have a problem. People who care about others make friends more easily.

- **Be friendly.** Smile when you see others. Show others that you are interesting and fun to be around, and they will want to be around you. Think about your body language and facial expressions. You can use your nonverbal communication skills, discussed in Chapter 5, to show that you are open to meeting people and that you are friendly. Also, make sure that you participate in whatever activities are going on around you if it's possible. That will show others that you are ready to be involved.

- **Be a good sport.** Be a team player. Make everyone feel like a winner. Don't worry about losing; just play the game as best as you can and have fun while doing it. In the next chapter, we will explain more about being a good sport.

- **Be interested.** Listen carefully to others and make them feel like what they have to say is important. Don't interrupt while they are talking.

- **Be flexible.** No one wants to hang out with or listen to someone who says or does the same things over and over again. Make sure you have new and different ideas to share that will be interesting to others. Remember to "Go with the flow" when someone else makes a suggestion.

- **Treat others the way you want to be treated.** If you want friends to treat you with respect and kindness, you need to make sure that you treat them with respect and kindness. Think carefully before you act or speak.

Unfriendly Behaviors

It's easy to make mistakes. **Sometimes you may do or say things that show you are not thinking about the perspectives of the people around you, even if you don't mean to.** For example, you might notice something different about a person who is near you. She could be wearing different clothes than you might expect or have a different hairstyle than she did the day before. Some people are overweight or have a visible handicap. You might observe these things and then want to talk about them because you noticed them. You might think that these are just factual observations, but the person you are speaking about might feel that you are being rude or unfriendly if you talk about them.

Suppose you meet someone from a country where it is traditional to wear a particular type of head covering that you haven't seen before. Saying something like, "Why are you wearing that? Nobody else is wearing that," will most certainly make the person feel very uncomfortable – particularly, if you say it out loud in front of other people. Whether the person is a stranger or someone you see every day, remember to think about what he or she might think if you say exactly what you want to, exactly at the moment you want to. It's like remembering the differences between "wanting to talk and needing to talk" (as discussed in Chapter 5) or paying attention to "personal or private topics" (also in Chapter 5).

Not thinking about others' point of view when speaking with them might hurt your chances of making and keeping friends. You might be someone who does some of these things without realizing it. If this happens to you, don't worry. You can always make a change when you make a mistake.

The following are examples of unfriendly behaviors that you should stay away from:

- **Being a bully.** Don't be mean and grouchy or threaten other kids, and don't be friends with mean and grouchy kids.

- **Being bossy.** Don't try to force kids to play what you want and follow your rules. Don't be mad when you don't get your way.

- **Being a name caller.** Don't say mean things about others. Don't try to make others really sad; no one likes to be called names.

- **Being a tattletale.** A tattletale is someone who tells an authority figure, like a teacher or parent, what other kids or even grownups are doing wrong. It's typical for kids to tell on other kids up until they are about 10 years old. Then they start to think more about what the other people around them are going to think if they "tell."

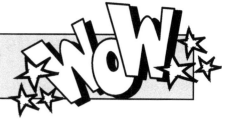

A good rule to remember is that you are only responsible for yourself first.

If a friend tells you that he decided to skip baseball practice to stay home and play video games, it is not your responsibility to tell the coach what you know. But there are times where you may hear something from a friend or acquaintance that makes you feel really uncomfortable. Things like cheating on a test, taking drugs, or someone getting hurt physically or emotionally either in school or in their home are private topics. If you feel uncomfortable with something that you have heard, you can go to an adult you trust and let them know you need help deciding whether to tell or not.

- **Being the "rule police."** Don't watch others to make sure they don't break the rules. In most instances, that is probably not your job. If a classmate decides to take out a novel to read, instead of the class textbook, that is his choice. You don't need to be responsible for anyone but yourself.

- **Being too silly.** Don't do silly things all the time or at the wrong time (in class, for example), even if other kids laugh. Sometimes it's fun to fool around in the classroom or to make jokes. But doing these kind of things over and over can bother others and maybe get them, or you, in trouble with a grownup. For more information on this, review the section on interrupting in Chapter 5 – Communication.

- **Being whiny.** Whining, or complaining, will not get you positive attention. No one wants to listen to someone complain all the time. Thinking positive can help prevent you from whining, as well as using an appropriate tone of voice to help you express yourself. Review the section on nonverbal communication and tone of voice in Chapter 5.

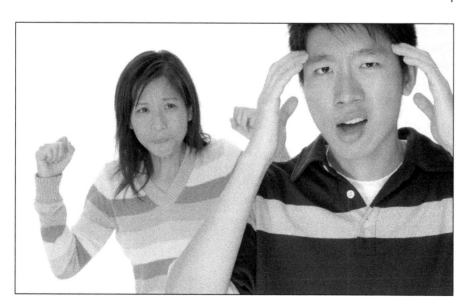

Keeping Friends

Most likely you will want to be around the friends you are close with, and you will take actions to keep them close to you.

If you are reading this book, you are old enough to take care of your friendships. If you have close friends, it is your responsibility, to your friends and to yourself, to keep them close to you. If you don't, your friends will notice that you aren't trying hard enough to keep the relationship going, and that might make them feel as if **you** are not a friend worth keeping.

In Chapter 4, we discussed understanding the thoughts and feelings of others. Understanding the points of view of others will help you a great deal when you are thinking about keeping your friendships going.

There are many things you can do to keep your friends close to you. You can:

- **Be honest.** Share your feelings appropriately if your friends are doing things that make you feel uncomfortable. Too much friendly teasing or not spending enough time together are things that sometimes happen that you might want to be honest about.

- **Be loyal and trustworthy.** Remember that the special things you share with your friends are important. Keep any secrets they might share with you, unless you think that your friend or someone else could be in danger. If you are unsure about whether a secret you've heard places someone in an unsafe situation, talk with a parent or another adult you trust so that they can help you figure it out.

- **Be supportive.** Your friends will want your attention and support when things are good for them and also when things are not going well for them. Learn to recognize these moments. Show your support by being there for them when they need it.

  For example, if they play sports, go to one of their games and cheer, or if they are performing in the school play, make sure you go to see it. Tell them afterward how proud you were of their performance. If a friend is going through a difficult time at home or in school, offer to do something that will help him solve the problem or take his mind off of it.

- **Remind your friends that their friendship is important to you.** You can do this by keeping promises, for example. If you promise a friend that you will go with her to see the new movie with your favorite actor, make sure you do it. If you change your mind, or go with someone else, she will definitely feel disappointed. Disappointing a friend over and over again shows that you don't care about the friendship or the person. If you seem to not care, the friend may decide not to be your friend any more.

Maintaining Friendships

In addition to the things already discussed, like remembering the "friendly behaviors" listed earlier in this chapter, and remembering your good communication and perspective-taking skills (see Chapters 4 and 5), there are other things you can do to help you keep your friendships with others.

- **Stay connected.** Computers are fun, and so are cell phones and PDAs. Today kids stay in touch through text messaging on their mobile phones, chatting on the computer, playing video games together on-line, or using social networking sites. These are great ways to stay in touch with your friends, to get information about them and learn about their thoughts, feelings, and interests.

  As long as you follow the rules that are set by your parents or a given website, and you're being **safe with your personal information,** such as not giving out your address or telephone number on the Internet or being very specific about what your daily routines are, you can use these things to help enhance your friendships and your social thinking skills. Just remember that technology is not a substitute for real interactions. It is a fun and different way to stay in touch. You must make moves to talk and spend time with your friends in person.

  Using the telephone is also a great way to stay connected. Almost everyone has a phone, and most people love to get calls. Don't be afraid of using the phone. If you want to have friends and get together and do things with them, you have to reach out. Learn how to use the phone appropriately to contact your friends and plan activities together.

- **Have fun.** If you are having friends over to your house, be prepared. Think about what you and your friend might like to do. Plan your time with your friend *before* they come over. Consult with your parents or whomever you need to when you are deciding on activities and make sure that they agree with your plan. Take care of any transportation that needs to be scheduled ahead of time.

- **Be a good host.** Having friends over to your house to hang out makes you the "host." It doesn't make you the "boss." Your job as the host is to make sure your guest feels comfortable. A good host …
  - Figures out something to do that everyone agress with
  - Avoids or quickly fixes arguments
  - Protects everyone's feelings from being hurt

- **Make good choices.** Think about the people you are choosing to hang out with. How do your parents or siblings feel about them? Are they responsible? Do they accept rules from authority figures? Do they make good choices when they pick friends to hang out with? Do they display the behaviors that a good friend would?

Use the people that you trust in your life to help you answer these questions. This will enable you to make better choices about who you are spending time with.

- **Get help if you have worries or concerns.** Sometimes friendships can be confusing. If you feel uncomfortable about anything that a friend is doing with you or saying to you, go to an adult that you trust and talk with them about it. Choosing to do this is a great start to good problem solving because they can help you figure out what is confusing to you and plan and organize what to say to your friend.

Big Picture Thinking About Relationships

Getting to know new people and staying in touch with the friends you have is important. Having positive relationships and successful friendships is a great goal. You need to use your perspective-taking and communication skills in order to do this.

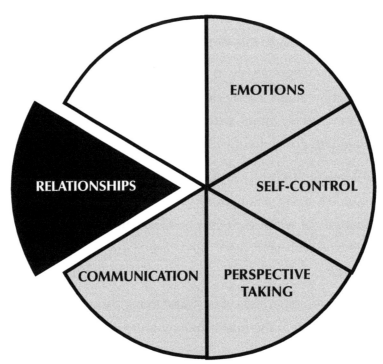

 KIDS IN ACTION REVIEW

The story example at the beginning of this chapter was about Angela and how she felt about meeting people at her new school. Her mom reminded her about the importance of paying attention to her nonverbal communication as well as other important details like perspective taking. When she was able to put all the clues together, Angela was successful at making new friends.

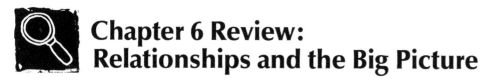

Chapter 6 Review:
Relationships and the Big Picture

In this chapter, you read about relationships. Being around other people in school, community activities, and sports often results in making connections that can become relationships that can eventually deepen into friendships. Having people around you with similar interests is fun. Even though you might not want to be with your friends all the time, try to stay connected so that you will be able to spend time with them when you want to.

Be aware of situations where you might meet new friends. Usually people have more than one good friend or best friend. Having groups of friends is also common. No matter how many friends you have, remember to display the kind of behaviors that attract friends – not the behaviors that make them turn away. Sometimes people feel like they might not want to make friends or find new friends. But the friendship "rules" are important for everyone. They apply to other situations also, like working in groups, which is something that everyone in school has to do sometimes. They are also important later in life on the job, for example.

 # Practice Ideas

1. **Honing Your Skills.** In order to make friends and be a good friend, you must be confident in yourself and your abilities. Use your journal to write about the qualities that you have that make you an interesting and special person. Show your list to an adult who can help you add to it.

2. **Friends Roster.** A roster is a usually a list of people who are grouped together in some way, like on a sports team or in a classroom. It's important to keep contact information about your friends so that you can get in touch with them for things like inviting them over to your house, checking on a homework assignment or getting a homework assignment if you forget yours, making plans for doing things together outside of school, or just checking in with them. You can use a regular address book, a computer-generated list, or the worksheet on page 146 (there is a blank one in the Appendix of this book on page A12) to help you gather the correct information and keep it current.

Friends Roster Example:

Name: Leslie Smith	Nickname: ?
Address: 6 Pine Drive Little Falls NJ 07424	Birthday: 2/13/2000
Home phone: 555-234-6175	Cell phone: 222-789-5678
Email: lsmithy@yahoo.com	Parents: Carla Fox and Steven Smith
Other family: Sister: Morgan; Dog: Cooper	
Interests: Soccer, swimming, drawing, playing the piano, singing	Friends you have in common: Harrison, Tracy, and Laurie W.
Things you enjoy doing together: Swimming at the town pool and water parks in the summer, doing craft projects, playing video games, watching movies	
Other information: Purple is her favorite color, and she loves Katy Perry's music	

3. **Acrostic.** Write an acrostic poem about yourself on a friendship topic. An acrostic poem uses the letters in a topic word to begin each line. All lines in the poem should relate to or describe the topic word. For example:

> **F** unny
>
> **R** espectful
>
> **I** nteresting
>
> **E** xtra special
>
> **N** ice
>
> **D** ependable

You can also use your name as the topic word. Here is an example using the name Cary:

> **C** urious
>
> **A** rtistic
>
> **R** esponsible
>
> **Y** oung man

4. **Journaling.** Use your journal to write about the friends you have. These entries can be your "friendly files." Write about some of the following:

- How did you meet?

- What did you think of each other when you first met?

- What do you have in common? What interests do you have that are different?

- What were some of your most fun experiences together?

- What do you hope to do together in the future?

If you don't currently have friends to whom this applies, try writing about what kind of friend you would like to have.

5. **Classified Ad**. Pretend you are advertising in a newspaper to find a new friend and write a classified advertisement. What would you write about yourself and what you are looking for so you would find the right kind of person? To make it more specific, you can write one ad for a "Friend" and one ad for a "Best Friend." How would these be different and how would they be the same?

6. **Lists.** Make a list of all the things you do alone. Look through the list and see if there are things that might be even more fun if you did them with a friend. Is there anything on your list that can't be done with a friend? If so, what?

7. **Reviewing "Friendly" and "Unfriendly" Behaviors.** Look back at the list of "friendly" and "unfriendly" behaviors on pages 141-142. Make a list of any "unfriendly" behaviors that you have problems with. Then show the list to someone else to see if they think your observations about your own behavior are correct. If not, list some ways that you might make changes in your behavior. You can use a chart like the one below to help you. You will find a blank copy in the Appendix on pages A13-A14.

Unfriendly Behavior	How It Makes Others Feel	What Can I Do to Make a Change?
Sometimes I engage in "silly" behaviors	Frustrated and annoyed	Practice better self-control
I sometimes forget to show interest in my friends	Left out, angry	Practice listening with interest to what friends have to say

8. **Relationship Pyramid.** In the Appendix on page A15, you will find a blank copy of the relationship diagram that was used in this chapter. The steps are labeled, but you need to add in the people in your life that fit into each step. Level 1 is you, so you would write in your name. Continue in that manner, adding as many names as you can to each level.

Chapter 7
The Big Picture: Interactions

In this chapter, we will discuss the skills you need to think about in order to get along with others and/ or interact with them. You interact with a lot of different people on a daily basis – family members, friends, and acquaintances. In order to have positive interactions with others, you need to think about things like:

- Sharing

- Working cooperatively in a group or as a team

- Being a good sport when playing games

- Being flexible when making decisions

- Joining in a group of people who are talking or playing together

- Accepting no

- Understanding how to deal with arguments

- Dealing with arguments with your friends

- Understanding how to share facts and opinions calmly with others

- Giving and receiving constructive criticism

- Giving compliments to others and receiving compliments politely

- Showing support for a friend

- Understanding the difference between friendly and mean teasing

- Understanding how to deal with teasing and bullying

These are just some of the things you need to think about. You also need to be aware of other people's thoughts and feelings by using your perspective-taking skills (remember Chapter 4!). Good communication skills (see Chapter 5) are another important part of getting along with others because you need to be able to express yourself clearly when speaking with the people you are working or playing with.

KIDS IN ACTION: INTERACTIONS

Santiago and Michael are in the sixth grade. They have been best friends since preschool. They live next door to each other, and their parents are close friends. Since they have grown up together and their parents are friends, they have always spent a lot of time hanging out together both at home and at school. It has never been difficult for them to find something to do together, but over the years, their interests have changed. Santiago is really involved in sports, such as soccer and kickball. He plays soccer on a travel team, which takes up a lot of his time after school and on weekends. Michael enjoys computers and science. He's thinking about joining the Chess Club at school.

With their new interests, the boys have had opportunities to meet other people and spend time with them. Santiago has become very friendly with many of the boys on his soccer team and he now has a much bigger group of friends. He hangs out with them a lot at school and on the weekends. Michael has met a few new people, but they don't spend a lot of time together outside of school, and the friendships have not developed into close relationships.

On weekends, when he wants to do something, Michael still expects Santiago to be available for him. He thinks that since they live next door to each other, they should still be "best friends" who spend a lot of time together. Michael doesn't always plan ahead and often just walks over to Santiago's house, rings the doorbell, and expects that he will be able to hang out. The past couple of times he has done this, Santiago has had some of his soccer friends over to practice in the backyard. Because he has known Michael for so long, Santiago has been friendly and invited him to join them. He specifically says to Michael ahead of time, "You are welcome to hang out with us, but we are working on some soccer skills in the backyard." Each time he has been invited, Michael has joined the group.

Even though Santiago has told Michael what the boys were going to be doing, it has still been difficult for Michael to fit in. He doesn't enjoy sports very much, and his soccer skills are not nearly as good as the other boys'. As a result, he usually spends most of his time watching, rather than playing, and he asks Santiago a lot of questions. Most of his questions are about when they are going to be able to switch to another activity. He interrupts Santiago and says things like, "Can we stop playing soccer now and do something on the computer instead? I have a new game I want to show you."

Santiago is becoming frustrated. Even though he tells Michael exactly what his plans are, Michael doesn't seem to understand that he will not be able to play computer games with him when his soccer friends are over. He explains to his dad, "I don't get it. I tell him exactly what's happening and then he ignores what I said. Why does he do that? I'm not inviting him over anymore ever."

Michael is feeling very left out. He explains to his mom, "Why does he invite me over and then ignore what I say? I tell him I want to do something different and he doesn't listen. He's not being fair."

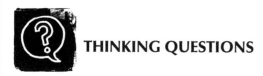

THINKING QUESTIONS

What is Santiago's problem? What is Michael's problem?

Santiago thinks that Michael is ignoring what he has said. Do you think that is true?

Michael thinks that Santiago isn't listening to him. Do you think that is true?

Is there a way that Santiago and Michael might be able to solve this problem?

Have you ever had a problem with a friend like this?

REWIND

It's not easy when friendships change. This is something that happens a lot as people get older and start to have different interests and goals. Santiago and Michael have a long-time friendship that seems to be changing. They may have to spend time together a little differently than before in order to accommodate that change, but it doesn't mean that they can't, or won't, be friends any more.

The pages in this chapter will help you understand the skills involved with social interactions and being a cooperative partner when you are with other people.

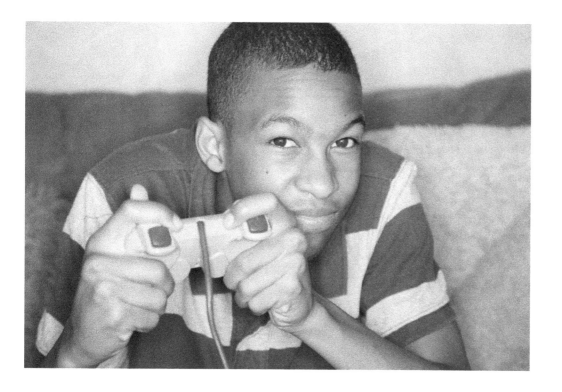

Sharing

Sharing is an important social skill. It shows people that you are friendly and caring, and it can also make you feel good about yourself.

You need to be fair when you share. **Sometimes "fair" means that everyone gets the same amount.** For example, if a friend wanted to share a snack with you, one person might suggest that the snack gets split evenly. This means that both people get the same amount. **Sometimes "fair" means the amount of something a person needs.** For example, in school, some students need more help than others. You might see your teacher giving extra help to a classmate on a test or a project that everyone is working on. It might seem "unfair" that someone would get more help than you on the same test or project, but in this case, it is fair because everyone gets what he or she really needs.

Sometimes "fair" is the amount a person has worked for and earned. For example, people who work together often have different jobs and different responsibilities. They also earn different salaries based on how much time they work and how big their responsibilities are. In this case, the money a person earns is related to the work that he or she does, which makes it fair for everyone.

When you aren't sharing at a time when you should be, others might think you are being "greedy."

Try not to be considered "greedy." Think about these important ideas:

- Understand that everyone deserves a fair share.

- Decide what is a fair share before you share something and let everyone decide what the fair way to share will be.

- Ask an adult to help if you and your friends cannot decide what a fair way to share is.

- Give others their share before you take yours.

- Don't take more than you should.

- Don't complain about what you get.

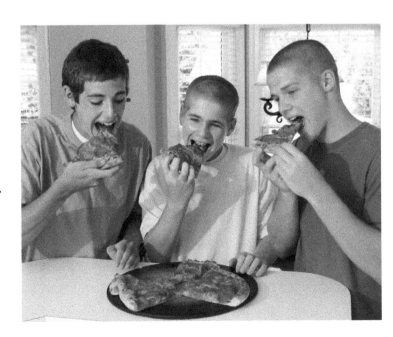

Being a Good Sport

Kids like to do things together because it's fun! Most kids know that having fun and being content with being a part of a group is what good sportsmanship is about.

If you are someone who is always arguing with other kids when you are playing with them, you are someone who is playing "to win at all costs." This means that you are only thinking about winning and aren't thinking about having fun. You also aren't thinking about the thoughts, feelings, and point of view of others.

Knowing how to be a good sport and trying to act like one will help you get along with others. Here are some specifics that you need to know.

A good sport …

Takes the game seriously and really wants to play. Don't "clown around" by doing things like stealing the ball and not giving it back.

Follows the rules of the game. Don't break the rules or change them to give yourself or your team an advantage.

Lets others have fun, too. Think about the other kids you are playing with and make sure that they are having a good time also. Stay in your position and wait your turn. Don't be a "ball hog" or try to take over the team. Don't try to play for other people.

Avoids arguments. Try not to get angry or fight with the people you are playing with. Don't play "referee" and tell other kids what they are doing wrong because that is the way arguments can start.

Always finishes the game. Stay until the end of the game even if you are tired or losing.

You can be a good sport if you …

- Are a good winner and a good loser
- Don't give up in the middle of a game because you don't like the way things are going
- Encourage other players – give compliments
- Don't tease the losers
- Play games because it's fun – not just to win

Teamwork/Cooperation

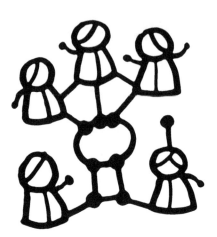

What does teamwork mean? The word says it all: **working together as a team.** Sometimes "team" really means team, like in sports, but sometimes a team is just a group of people you are working or playing with.

The Big Picture here is that you are trying to work well with others. This includes things like:

- **Taking turns.** Make sure that everyone in the group gets a turn to share their ideas or do some of the work. Remember that everyone wants to be a part of the group activities.

- **Being a good sport.** Even though we say "Be a good sport," this doesn't have to do only with sports or games. Good sportsmanship is important for any kind of teamwork, so remember to keep those rules in mind.

- **Sharing.** This means sharing "things," like materials or equipment, and also sharing ideas with others and accepting their ideas in a way that will be helpful to the group.

- **Being fair.** You just read about what it means to be "fair." Make sure everyone in your group gets to have a fair share in what you are doing.

- **Thinking about others.** Don't forget your perspective-taking skills. Being aware of and alert to other people's feelings, needs, and intentions is important if you are working in a group.

- **Manners.** Remember to be friendly and polite when working with others. Don't forget that people expect you to follow the social rules of the situation you are in. Chapter 5 includes a lot of information about good manners for conversations with others.

- **Communication.** Use your listening skills and pay attention to what others are saying and doing. Stay involved by talking with the others in your group and make sure that they receive the correct verbal and nonverbal messages from you. This may be a good time to review Chapter 5, which contains important information about nonverbal communication and conversation skills.

Joining In

"**Joining in**" means you want to get together with others who are already in a group "doing something."

You can join into a conversation with other kids who are already talking together. This was discussed in Chapter 5. You can also join in with kids who are already working or playing together.

Since the group has already started without you, it is not completely "open" to you. How you speak and act when you begin to join in is an important part of whether the group chooses to let you stay.

Joining in is a process. It usually doesn't happen right away. You need to take certain steps so others will view what you do and say in a positive way. You need to think about how others will respond to you when you try to join a group.

People usually respond well if you approach slowly and show an interest in them and the activity they are involved in.

Just because you want to join a group doesn't mean that the group has to allow you to join. There are many reasons why a group might not "open up" to another person. In Chapter 5, "Joining Into a Conversation" was discussed. The following pages in this chapter talk about steps you might take if you want to try to join with others who are already working or playing together. Whether it involves talking together or working/playing together, the two types of situations are similar. There are also pages about why some groups might say "no" and how you can deal with that. However, if you use the "joining in" steps and view the whole situation, you will have a better chance of getting a "yes" answer to your request to join in.

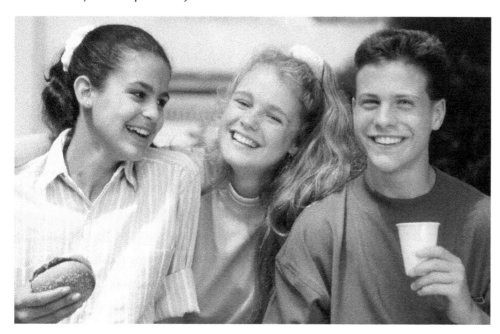

Joining a Game ... 1, 2, 3

Here are the steps you should use to join in to a game or activity with others:

1. **Get closer and watch.** Stand near the group and carefully watch the others first. Being a good observer before you get involved in the game or activity is important. This also shows others that you are interested.

2. **Gather information.** Make sure that you know the game the kids are playing. Getting in with a group of kids who are already playing is easier if you know the game ahead of time. Wanting to learn a new game is a great idea, but most times when kids are already playing, they are not able to help you enough so that you can learn. You might have to wait until there is a break, or a new game starting.

   Check the "skills" of the other kids, too. For example, if you know how to play basketball and you see some kids at the playground involved in a game, you might want to join in because you like it and know how to play. But if the kids who are playing have skills that are more advanced than yours, you might want to wait until there is a group that you will match better with.

3. **Make comments.** When you decide you are ready to join in, making a comment or saying something nice to the other kids who are playing shows them that you are interested. You can say things like, "Nice shot" or "You're really great at that game." If your comment is heard, the group will probably "open up" to respond to you.

   If the group opens up in response to your comment or compliment, you can take that as an opportunity to ask to join in. You might say something like, "Can I play in the next game?" or "Can I play the winner?" depending on what kind of game or activity is happening.

4. **Wait for a pause.** If the group does not open up in response to your comments, you can wait for a pause in the game and then ask to join in. Say something like, "Can I play the next game?" or "Do you think I could play, too?" Most of the time boys ask to join the "side" or team that needs help, like the "losing side" or the team with fewer players. Girls usually ask the girl who "owns" the jump rope or ball or the one who made up the game.

5. **Accept no for an answer.** Being turned down from games by other children is a fact of life. Everyone gets turned down sometimes. Kids who are successful socially get turned down, but it doesn't upset them. Expect to be turned down at least about half the time you try to join others. Be prepared to hear "no" and remember that it shouldn't be a big deal. Just **"Go with the flow;"** try not to cause problems for the people who are already playing or working together. And **think flexibly**, look for another group of people who are doing something you find interesting and give it another try.

Why Do Kids Say No?

Getting "turned down" from games is a fact of life. Sometimes kids will tell you why they are saying no and other times they won't. But here are some common reasons why kids say no when you ask to join in.

- **Trying to join in the wrong way.** Maybe you didn't ask to join in the right way. Don't forget that joining in is a process. That means there is more than one step that you need to remember.

- **Past experiences.** Maybe there is something that you did to the kids before, like avoiding them or getting them into trouble with a teacher. Or maybe they remember a time when you played with them and it didn't go so well.

- **Incompatibility.** Maybe the kids you tried to join aren't interested in the same things you are. They could be kids that are too "athletic" and your ideas and thoughts about what they are doing are too different from theirs.

- **Not interested.** The kids you chose might not want to meet new friends. Even though that might sound strange, it is a possibility.

- **Misunderstandings.** The kids might have misunderstood what you wanted to do. Maybe they didn't feel like playing with you right then.

If you think that one of the above is the reason why you have been turned down, you can try to do something about it. Here are some ideas …

- If you think you joined in the wrong way, make sure that next time you follow the joining in "rules." Watch first and praise other kids. Wait for a pause in the action and then ask to join.

- If you think that someone has a problem with you because of something that happened before, make sure to remember that you should treat others as you would like them to treat you. Choose a different group of kids that you know you can get along with.

- If you think that the children you chose have interests or skills that are different from yours, pick other children who are closer to your skill level and interests.

- If you think that they just aren't interested in meeting new people, pick other kids to join in with.

- If you think they said no because they misunderstood you, state your request to join differently. For example, maybe you weren't clear with your words, so rephrase them. Or maybe you need to be more specific, so point out to them that you noticed they have two less kids on a team.

Remember, everyone gets turned down some time. Expect that it will happen some of the time to you, too. Being prepared and being able to move on will help you get motivated to find another group of children who will say yes.

Accepting No for an Answer

So now you know that kids say no sometimes and you know that it is important to be able to deal with this. The Big Picture here is: Take "no!" for an answer and move on. This means you need to "go with the flow" and make different choices.

If you ask to join a group of kids and are not successful, here are some steps you can take after that will help you move on.

Step 1 – Listen carefully

- Look at them to show them that you are paying attention.

- Don't stare, make faces, or look away.

- If you are upset, control your feelings. Try to relax and stay calm.

- Listen carefully; this will help you understand what the person is saying (not talking is the best way to listen).

Step 2 – Respond appropriately

- Let them know that you heard them and that you understand what they are saying.

- If you are asked a question, answer right away and speak clearly.

- Don't sound angry or start to argue. This can cause problems.

Step 3 – Stay in control of your emotions

- You might be feeling angry, disappointed, or frustrated. Remember that people notice how you deal with those feelings.

- Staying calm shows that you are serious about the situation and that you can have control in a difficult moment.

- Showing anger or frustration in a way that hurts or annoys others can make the situation worse.

Step 4 – Getting more information

- If you aren't sure about why you weren't allowed to join in, you can try and ask the person later. Or, if you need to, you can explain the situation to an adult that you trust. He or she may be able to help you approach the other child, or even just talk with you about the situation so that you can understand it better and learn something for next time.

- Take some time to relax and think. Think about what you might want to say to the person who told you "no."

- Plan what you are going to say before you say it.

- Accept the answer that they give you, and make sure to thank the person for listening to you again.

Remember that how you act this time will affect what will happen next time. If you don't accept no in an appropriate way, other kids will remember how you acted, and they may not want to hang out with you in the future.

Important Things to Remember *Before* You Start Playing a Game

Sometimes kids get very involved with the details of a game and forget that the main reason for playing a game is to have fun.

Before you get started, it's important to remember what to do in the following situations.

- **Winning and losing.** No matter how good you are at something, sometimes you win and sometimes you lose. You never know what is going to happen when you start a game; you have to finish in order to find out. Don't take winning or losing a game too seriously.

- **Who goes first?** You might think that going first in a game will give you a special advantage over your opponent. This isn't always true. Sometimes it's better to go second, or last. Just know that you can't always go first because it's important to take turns. There are easy ways to decide who is going to go first: age, alphabetically, rolling the dice, or spinning the spinner. Be fair about getting started.

- **Running out of time.** Sometimes you can't finish the game because there is not enough time to play until someone wins or if the game ends in a tie. Be prepared for this by knowing right from the beginning that you might not be able to finish what you have started. **Thinking flexibly** (see Chapter 3 – "black-and-white" vs. "rainbow thinking") will help you find solutions to these kinds of problems.

- **Being choosy.** You may not always be able to get your first choice when it comes to deciding what game to play, what color playing piece you want, or what name your team agrees upon. Usually, kids decide these things together in a way that is fair to everyone. These are small details that don't make a big difference in the outcome of a game or in how much fun you are going to have.

Always remember to be a good sport no matter what. Be flexible and be prepared to lose or win. Having fun should be your main goal.

Fact vs. Opinion

Facts are statements that can be proven and that do not change. For example, "The movie *Despicable Me* opened on July 9, 2010."

Opinions are statements that say something about how you or someone else thinks or feels about a situation. Opinions might change over time, and different people often have different opinions. For example, a statement like "I thought the movie *Despicable Me* was the best movie that Disney ever made" is an example of an opinion.

Sharing opinions can help add to a conversation. You need to be respectful of other people's opinions and share your own in an appropriate way so that you don't make other people feel uncomfortable. The following can help you do this.

- **Remember to apply the rules of conversation** that you read about in Chapter 5.

- **Remember that statements of opinion include words like *think, feel, believe, always, never, none, most, least, best,* and *worst*.** All of your opinions should be stated like this. A good example is something like, "I believe there is no reason to go to any other grocery store because Stop n' Shop is the most convenient."

- **Keep in mind that fact statements don't have anything to do with what people think or feel about things.** They are easily proven, like "Today is Saturday." In a case like this, you could look it up on a calendar to find out if it were true or not.

- **Allow other people to share their opinions on a topic.** They may feel differently about something than you do and that's acceptable.

- **Don't force your opinions on others.** Don't talk too much about the same idea. No one has to think exactly the same things that you do.

- **Don't try to make your opinions sound like facts and don't accept it when others do it.** Sometimes people want you to think the same way that they do. They might try to do this by making their opinions and thoughts sound like they are facts. For example, if a friend doesn't like a movie you selected, he might say something like, "I read on the Internet that 90% of the people that saw that movie didn't like it at all."

    It's not fair for someone else to try to force their opinions on you in that way. And it is not fair for you to force your opinions on someone else. Everyone should be able to form their own opinions and share them with others appropriately.

- **Know the difference between facts and opinions** so that you can better understand what someone else is talking about. Look things up or ask others if you are not sure.

Arguments

Everyone is different, and different people think differently, or have different opinions (ideas) about situations and other things. Sometimes having different opinions and thoughts can lead to disagreements, especially if one person feels very strongly about something.

When people get "stuck" with their differing opinions, and communication becomes difficult, or angry, we might say that the discussion has turned into an argument.

On the next few pages you will read more about arguments and how you should respond in those situations.

Arguments at Home

At home you might get into an argument with your brothers or sisters, mother, father, step-parents, or even grandparents.

Sometimes arguing happens a lot with one particular family member, like a brother or sister, or maybe you only argue with a family member every once in a while. With whom, when, and how much you argue with family members may depend on how often you see them or how different your opinions and thoughts are from theirs.

Occasional disagreements and arguments with brothers and sisters will happen. Parents and other adults in charge at home understand this. When an argument or fight happens, siblings sometimes need help from an adult member of the family to get things worked out. At other times, the kids can fix it themselves.

Suppose there is only one computer in your house that you and your sister have to share. Maybe you come home from school one day wanting to use the computer to visit your favorite website, but your sister is already using the computer.

You need to figure out how to get a turn. If talking about the problem doesn't help, and if you can't agree on what to do, you may need help from an adult. When arguments go on for a long time, and it is too hard for the people involved to reach a compromise, it is best to ask for help.

Constant arguing between siblings is usually not acceptable. It can be difficult for parents to see their children fighting all the time, and they might feel frustrated. They may also become annoyed or frustrated with their children if they have to help them stop arguing all the time. You will probably see your mom or dad get upset or angry when this happens.

At home, adults make the rules and the schedule, and children may disagree with their choices or ideas. Expressing disappointment or disagreeing with an adult is okay, as long as you express those feelings appropriately through discussion.

It's important that you try to understand the adult's point of view in the situation (see Chapter 4 on perspective taking). Knowing when the conversation about the disagreement is over is also very important. If you go on and on, it may seem like you are arguing, which makes things more difficult for yourself and others.

For example, suppose your parents have told you that you can't watch a certain television show because they think it is not appropriate for kids your age. Maybe you are disappointed because a lot of your friends watch the show. You try to talk to your parents about it, and they tell you they aren't going to change their minds any time soon, so you should stop talking about it. If you keep bringing it up over and over again, you might make your parents angry and find yourself dealing with the consequences of their anger, which could include a punishment, depending on the rules in your home.

These rules about arguing at home are not just limited to your parents. They are true for any grown-up that is in charge in your home, including a babysitter.

Arguments in School

You "carry" your opinions and thoughts with you everywhere, including school. Having different opinions can result in disagreements or arguments. It's easy to get into an argument with someone if you are not open to hearing what they have to say.

At school, students may get into arguments with other students; this is expected, as long as it does not turn into a physical fight. Students may also disagree with teachers, assistant teachers, aides, the principal, or any other grownup at school. The teacher (or other grownup in charge) is responsible for making the rules, assignments, and activities. This means that they can also change their minds about the rules, assignments and activities.

Students may express their opinions as long as it is done appropriately and at the right time.
For example, suppose your teacher decides to change the date of a test. During class she announces that the test will take place next week, instead of two weeks away. You might feel angry or frustrated by this decision, but calling out and arguing with the teacher in the middle of class is not the right way to let her know how you feel. Find a time to speak to the teacher privately, plan what you will say, be ready to accept no for an answer, and move on.

No matter what, students should be aware of when the discussion is over and be prepared to move on. That is, you will need to accept "no" and move on. Not recognizing this moment can cause further problems.

A student may be given consequences for arguing with other students, and especially with adults at school. Any further arguing about the consequences will not help you get out of the punishment. **Understand that once an argument has reached a point where you are receiving consequences, it is no use to continue the argument.**

If a student gets into an argument with a teacher or another grownup in charge at school, she is usually expected to apologize. A lot of times, this means that the student is asked to write a letter or to see the teacher in person and let the teacher know she is sorry about what has happened. Whether you want to or not, it is important to make an apology that the teacher will accept. Say you are sorry, and move on.

Disagreements or differing opinions don't always have to turn into a huge argument. There are appropriate ways to talk about a problem, or negotiate, when you are having a problem with another person, and there are generally solutions to problems that will make everyone feel comfortable, called a compromise. You will read about these next.

Negotiation and Compromise

Negotiating refers to the talking that people do when they are trying to resolve an argument. It involves gathering the thoughts and opinions of everyone involved and working on an agreement that will make everyone involved feel comfortable.

Compromise refers to an agreement that is reached through discussion. A compromise is reached when everyone involved in the argument is able to decide what an acceptable solution is in order to move forward. Making a compromise usually involves one or more people accepting something different than they originally thought they wanted.

Let's look at an example. Suppose you have invited a friend over to your house to hang out and watch a movie. Once he arrives, you suggest a movie that you have been hoping to see. But your friend doesn't like your idea and suggests something different that you aren't interested in. The discussion you are having about what to watch is a **negotiation.**

Since you have both made suggestions that have been rejected, you need to come up with a new idea, or else you will have nothing to do. That is, you will need to come up with a **compromise:** an idea that will be fair enough and make both of you feel satisfied with the decision. Maybe your friend says something like, "Let's watch my choice first, and then we can watch yours." If you agree on this option, it means that you won't be seeing your movie right away, but you will get a turn. And so will your friend.

Reaching a compromise isn't always easy, because you might have to give something up. In the example above, you don't get to have what you want immediately, but you will get it eventually. On the other hand, if you decided together that it would be better to watch a completely different movie, you would have to give up your idea altogether and watch your movie another time.

Usually a lot of different ideas are shared when you are negotiating a compromise. Listening to all of them is a good idea.

It is important to be able to negotiate and make compromises when you have disagreements with others, especially with your friends. **When you have close relationships with your friends, being with them is always what's most important, not what you are doing together.**

Constructive Criticism

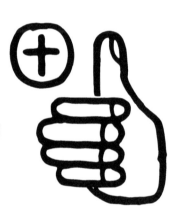

Constructive criticism is telling others, in a supportive way, something that will help them improve something about themselves or something they have done. Constructive criticism highlights both negative and positive points, but it is never meant to be insulting to the person to whom it is directed.

The following skill steps will help you to remember how to give and accept constructive criticism.

Steps for Giving Constructive Criticism

1. Look at the person and use a pleasant tone of voice.

2. Begin with a positive statement like, "I know you've been working really hard at playing that game ..."

3. Be specific and tell why this is a problem or is otherwise unsatisfactory or unacceptable, "But you might do better if you remembered to use your 'wild card.'"

Steps for Accepting Constructive Criticism

1. Remember that the person is trying to help you. Don't take it personally.

2. Listen carefully to the suggestion and the reasons why it may be important to change.

3. Thank the person for the suggestion and then decide if you want to follow it.

Compliments

A compliment is an expression of praise, congratulation, or encouragement. You can give compliments to others, both verbally and nonverbally (like in writing or with gestures), and you can accept compliments from others.

When you give a compliment in the appropriate way, you can make other people feel great about themselves. And getting a compliment and accepting it with confidence can make you feel good about yourself.

Here are some important things to remember about the Big Picture when giving compliments:

- **Sincerity.** You give compliments to show others that you are thinking about them and their feelings. Compliments should come from your heart, and you should really mean them.

- **Audience**. Who are you planning to give a compliment to? For example, as a student, you wouldn't want to compliment your principal or teacher on doing their job well. Because you are younger, you don't have enough experience to make those kinds of statements. Instead, stick to letting them know how much you enjoyed the activities or lessons they have planned for you.

- **Perspective.** As we discussed in Chapter 4, think about how others will think and feel about the compliment you want to give them.

- **Timing.** Choose the right time to give a compliment. Is the person ready to listen, or are they in the middle of doing something with somebody else? Will you be talking about something that other people can hear also, or is it better to share the compliment privately?

  Compliments are like "topics" – some are universal, some are particular, and some are private. Review the section in Chapter 5 to help you remember the information on topics. You can also read the section following this about "inside and outside compliments" to help you get a better idea about what kinds of compliments people give and receive.

- **Choice of words.** Not everything you think about someone is a compliment. For example, you might think that the color of someone's skin is beautiful, but if you said so the person might misunderstand your intention and think that you are drawing attention to racial differences. In this example, instead of drawing attention to "skin color," which might be misunderstood, it might be better to say something general like, "I love the color of your outfit today; it really makes you look pretty."

Here are the skill steps to remember about giving and receiving compliments:

Steps for Giving a Compliment

1. Look at the person you want to compliment.

2. Speak clearly.

3. Be specific about what you like.

4. Use positive words.

5. Wait for the person to respond to your compliment.

Steps for Accepting a Compliment

1. Look at the person who is complimenting you.

2. Thank the person for the compliment in a kind way. Say something like, "Thanks for noticing" or "That was so nice of you to say." This let's the person know that you heard what she said and that you are happy that she made an effort to talk to you.

"Outside" and "Inside" Compliments

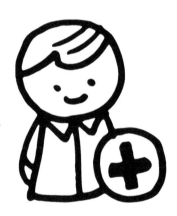

You can compliment people on things about their appearance or on things you observe them doing. These are things we can "see" about the person; we can call them "outside" compliments. You can also compliment people on things that have to do with their personality traits or things we know about them as we get to know them more personally but that we cannot actually see. These are "inside" compliments.

Outside Compliments

Usually these are things that we can see like haircuts, clothes, etc. Other things that would fall in the category of "outside" compliments include making a great catch at a baseball game or performing well in a play. These kinds of compliments are easy to give to anyone, whether we know them well or not. They can also be great conversation starters.

"Inside" Compliments

These are compliments about something in a person that you can't necessarily "see." It is usually a comment or a personality trait, like "You're really nice" or "You're a great friend." These are things you can say about a person that you have gotten to know well or to someone you consider a close friend. Getting to know about someone's "inside" qualities takes some time, and has to do with how well you know them.

Teasing

There are different types of teasing. **Sometimes teasing is friendly, but at other times it is meant to be mean. It is important to know the difference.**

Friendly Teasing

This is when someone gives you a "hard time" about something but does it in a nice or humorous way. For example, maybe you are someone who loves *Harry Potter*. You show other kids how much you love the books by talking about them all the time, watching the movies over and over, and reading the books in your free time at school. All of the close friends in your "inner circle" know that this is your "thing," or your interest. They sometimes joke with you by saying things like, "So where did you park your broom today?" You can tell by their words and tone of voice that the jokes are meant to be funny, and you probably laugh along with them.

This kind of teasing is done to make you laugh, not to hurt your feelings. Someone you know well usually does it, and you trust the person wouldn't purposefully hurt your feelings. Most important, you should understand that it is a joke, laugh with them, and not feel upset by it.

Mean Teasing

This is when someone gives you a hard time about something and is trying to hurt your feelings or make you feel bad about yourself. Think about our *Harry Potter* example. Suppose someone you don't know well also notices that you like the *Harry Potter* books. Maybe they don't understand you or your interests very well and when they see you they make comments like, "So, did you ride your broom to school today, witch?" in a nasty tone of voice. You can tell by their choice of words and nonverbal communication (as discussed in Chapter 5) that they are **intentionally** trying to be mean.

You can tell that this is mean teasing because you don't think it's funny and you feel uncomfortable and sad. Mean teasing may happen repeatedly, and someone you don't know very well usually does it.

Dealing With Teasing

We just talked about how to tell if you are dealing with "friendly teasing" or "mean teasing." After you have decided what kind of teasing it is, you can do the following:

1. **If it's friendly teasing,** you can go along with the teasing and be a good sport about it. Remember, friendly teasing shouldn't make you feel upset or hurt. If a good friend thinks that he is teasing you in a friendly way and you don't like it, you need to let him know that your

feelings have been hurt and that you want him to stop. If he is a real friend, he will respect your feelings, apologize, and stop the teasing.

2. **If it's mean teasing**, you can:

- Ignore the teasing or the person who is doing it.

- Tell the person to stop in an assertive way. This means you make yourself clear by using direct statements with appropriate nonverbal communication (stern tone of voice and serious facial expressions, for example).

- Walk away from the situation.

- Tell a grownup who you think can help you.

- Just say, "So what?" Making a comment like this shows that you don't care.

- Use humor as a defense.

- Use a calming strategy to make sure you can stay in control (see Chapter ?).

When you deal with teasing appropriately, others will respect you.

Bullying

Bullying is a serious and difficult problem. And it is unacceptable! Sometimes you might want to believe that it is a small problem, but it is a really big problem. It might be that a person threatens or makes fun of you every once in a while, or it might be a continuous thing, where the bully has a deliberate plan to make you feel humiliated on a regular basis.

A serious problem with a bully can be:

- When someone is **repeatedly** pressuring you or threatening you to do something you don't want to do.

- When someone is **repeatedly** doing something that makes you feel angry, afraid, upset, frustrated, humiliated, or embarrassed.

- Physical, verbal, nonverbal, or a combination of these.

- When someone ignores, isolates, or doesn't include you on a regular basis.

Even someone you think is supposed to be a friend can bully you. It doesn't matter who is doing the bullying; it must be stopped.

It is common for kids to want to deal with bullying on their own, **BUT** most times, it is too challenging for them to handle alone. If you are being bullied, act quickly and go to an adult you trust. In most instances, this is the best and sometimes, the only way, to stop it from continuing. Asking for help dealing with a bully can be hard for kids because:

- They feel too humiliated or embarrassed to talk about it.

- They feel that no one will understand or believe them.

- They feel that if they try to get help it will make the bullying worse.

Even if you feel these things, you must ask for help. Talk to an adult you trust at school or at home and let him or her know what is happening and how you are feeling. Let the adult help you by taking charge and "tattling" on the bully. The adult should be able to do this in private, in a way that will not call attention to you or your problem. The adult can also help you get some "protection" from the bully, like changing seats or classes at school if necessary.

Bullies like kids who go along with whatever they say. Remember, it is better NOT to do what the bully wants you to do. You don't have to fight; just don't give the bully any kind of control over you. Get away from the bully and go to an adult if possible. Don't worry about being called names if you run, getting away from a bully is a smart thing to do.

Make sure that you hang out with your close friends. Spend time with them. Kids who are with friends and not alone are less likely to be bullied. And if you need it, your real friends will be there to help you find a way out of a problem situation and also they will stick up for you.

Remember ... Bullies can only **try** to bully you. They are only successful if you **let them** bully you.

You are in charge of your thoughts, feelings, and behavior. If you don't let their words or actions affect your feelings in a negative way, then they have not been successful with their teasing. A bully or teaser wants to see your reaction, so don't give them any and follow the suggestions given above.

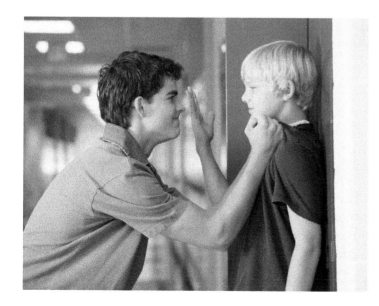

Big Picture Thinking About Interactions

Getting along with others includes all the things that help you make and keep friends. Things like being a good sport, compromising with others, being agreeable, joining in, dealing with teasing and bullying, and accepting "no" are just some of the topics that we discussed in this chapter.

Using perspective-taking skills to understand what others are thinking and feeling (see Chapter 4) is another important part of getting along with others. In addition, you need to communicate effectively with others so that they understand your thoughts, feelings, and ideas (see Chapter 5).

Getting along with others is an area that might challenge your ability to manage difficult emotions. Therefore, displaying self-control (Chapter 3) when you are feeling upset by your interactions with others is very important.

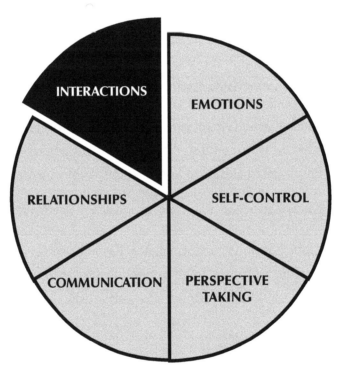

 KIDS IN ACTION REVIEW

At the beginning of the chapter, you read the story of Santiago and Michael and how changes in their friendship were making it difficult for them to get along. Both Michael and Santiago need to understand each other's feelings about the situation and work out a better way to communicate with each other in order to solve this problem.

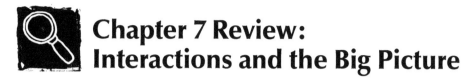

Chapter 7 Review:
Interactions and the Big Picture

Although friends usually have common interests and enjoy doing things together, they can still disagree. Be sure to remember that. Disagreements can usually be resolved with a compromise, which involves each person "giving" a little bit or being more flexible than he or she might really want to be.

You don't have to get along with everyone all of the time. There will always be people who might make you feel discouraged, but you need to view the situation as a whole in order to know how to deal with it properly.

 # Practice Ideas

1. **Positive Self-Talk.** In this chapter, we talked about a lot of situations where you might need to deal with difficult emotions. Planning ahead so that you can deal with these moments is very important. Practice your positive self-talk (see Chapter 3) to help you out. Positive statements you can say to yourself include:

   - "I have the power to succeed in everything I do."

   - "I only have positive thoughts about myself and others."

   - "I feel good about myself and accept me as I am."

   - "I can handle any situation with ease."

   Make a list of positive statements in your journal or on index cards where they are handy for when you want to look at them. Repeating these types of statements to yourself will help you live them.

   On the next page is the beginning of a worksheet (you can find the whole worksheet in the Appendix on page A16) designed to help you go further with positive self-talk. You can use the worksheet to look more in depth at situations where you did not focus on positive thoughts. These can be situations you are in on a regular basis where you know it's difficult for you to stay positive. For example, maybe you always hate gym class because you have a hard time with sports and you have difficulty staying positive.

"Walking in the Positive" Worksheet

What Is/Was the Situation?	How Are/Were You Feeling?	What Are/Were You Thinking?	Change Your Negative Thoughts to Positive Thoughts
Didn't understand the math homework	Stressed, angry, overwhelmed	I am bad at math and never get things right	I will remember that I try really hard at math and there are lots of other things that I am good at

2. **Point of View Role-Play.** Review your perspective-taking skills (see Chapter 4). Understanding the thoughts, feelings, and intentions of others is an important skill. Thinking about the point of view of all the people involved in a situation is the key to opening a lot of closed doors. After you have reviewed, it is time to practice. Find a partner to help you, like a parent or another adult. With the list of problem-solving situations below, take the perspective of one of the characters and role-play what they might say in the situation described.

- *Meg and Nancy are best friends.* They always go to the mall on Saturdays and browse the stores, even when they don't have money to buy anything. Today, Meg wants to do something different. She heard that a bunch of kids from school are going to a carnival in a nearby town, and she thinks it would be fun. Meg needs to tell Nancy about her idea, but she is a little worried that Nancy won't like it.

- *Lucas and Liana are close friends.* They eat lunch together pretty much every day at school. After they finish eating, Lucas always asks Liana to buy him an extra snack. Even though Liana doesn't like to do it, she usually does. Finally one day, Liana decides that she doesn't want to buy extra snacks for Lucas any more, and she needs to let him know that he has to bring his own money from now on.

- *You are watching your favorite television show on Sunday morning and the TV suddenly goes blank right in the middle.* Your parents have worked hard all week, and they are still sleeping. You want to go and wake them up to help you fix it.

- *You are eating dinner in a restaurant with your family when you spot a famous sports star enter the restaurant with his family.* The hostess seats him at the table next to you. You really want to ask him for his autograph.

- *Pretend you are a parent.* Your child has saved about $100.00 from her allowance and doing some work in the neighbor's yard. She wants to spend all of the money she has earned at the amusement park and you don't think it's a good idea.

- ***Chamil and Karim are planning to go to the movies together.*** Chamil's mom tells him that she will give him $20.00 to go to the movies after he mows the lawn. Before he is finished, his mom goes to the store and doesn't get back in time to give him the money before they have to leave for the movie theater. Chamil tells Karim that he knows his mom keeps some extra money in the cookie jar in the kitchen, but he doesn't know if he should take it without asking first. Karim encourages Chamil to take the money and replace it later without telling his mom. Chamil thinks maybe they should wait for his mom to return and go to a later movie.

3. **Making a Plan to Join In.** Think about a time during your day when you might want or need to join in with others. Some suggestions:

   - Joining in a game at recess

   - Finding a group to sit with at lunchtime

   - Getting into a group conversation in the hallway, classroom, or other setting in school

   - Finding a partner, or partners, for a group activity in class

   - Joining a team in gym

   - Getting together with a group to "hang out" after school

   Choose a situation that is familiar to you, one that you might have experienced before. Once you have decided, put your plan into action. Think about the steps for joining in that were discussed in this chapter (see page 158) and try them out. Decide what you will do if you are given a "no" answer (see pages 159-160).

4. **Friendly Teasing.** Try to remember times where someone teased you in a friendly way. Answer these questions:

   - Who is the person and what is his relationship to you?

   - What was the "teasing" about?

   - How did you know it was friendly teasing?

   - Did you react appropriately?

   Friendly teasing is a part of growing up and having close friends. As long as the teasing doesn't hurt your feelings or happen on a continual basis, it's something that you will need to learn to deal with.

5. **"Bullies Can Only Bully You If You Let Them."** Think about this statement. What does it really mean? This could be a good conversation to have with an adult you know and trust. It also makes a very good journal entry "starter."

6. **"I feel ..." Statements.** Being assertive without being mean is critical. It's important to let others know how we feel and give them a reason why their behavior is making us feel a certain way. We also want to let them know how we want the situation to be different. Using "I feel ... " statements may help us get more positive results with all kinds of teasing, criticism, and arguments. Here are examples of "I feel ..." statements:

   - "I feel really uncomfortable when you sit so close to me. Could you remember to leave some space in between us next time?"

   - "It hurts my feelings when you tease me about my glasses. I know you are doing it in a friendly way, but I am hoping that you can find another way to have fun with me."

   - "I really felt excluded when you invited Hayley and Marisa to go to the mall last Saturday. Maybe next time I could come, too?"

   - "I know you are trying to be helpful, but I would really like to try to get this done by myself. I will ask you if I need your help."

   - "I feel that it is unfair when you don't let me play basketball with you at recess. Maybe next time you could try to include me?"

   Think about the "I feel ..." statements above and create some more. Relate them to situations that you have experienced and role-play some of the examples as practice.

7. **Constructive Arguments.** Argue with a purpose and know when to back down. Role-play some arguments with a partner. Having two people involved in the role-play is helpful because each "player" can take a different position in the disagreement scenarios below.

   - You and a friend want to go to the movies and she is refusing to see the movie that you want to see.

   - A good friend falsely accuses you of stealing money out of her backpack.

   - You're going to a friend's house and your parents want you home for dinner. You want to stay later.

   - A teacher thinks you were distracting the class by talking too much. You know you weren't the only one.

   - You want to buy a new video game but your parents think it's too violent. Everyone else your age has it already.

While you are role-playing, think about the argument you are having and who you are arguing with. Is this an argument where you might have to use your words to convince someone that your way might be better? Is this an argument with a person that you need to treat with respect? Is this a situation where you might actually be able to change someone else's perspective? Do you know when to end the argument? After the role-play, fill out the checklist below (find a blank in the Appendix on page A17) for each situation.

Constructive Arguments Worksheet

Did I …	Remember to be critical of ideas and not people?	Let everyone have a chance to share their thoughts?	Listen attentively to the other person's ideas?	Focus on making the best possible decision for everyone?	Generate multiple solutions to the problem and reach an appropriate agreement?
Role-Play #1 Meg and Nancy	Yes	I had difficulty with interrupting	I had difficulty with interrupting	Yes	I came up with 3 possibilities

Chapter 8

Getting the Big Picture!

I n the first chapter of this book, learning to get the Big Picture in a social situation was discussed. This means that you are looking at the "whole" situation and not focusing only on the details that are happening right at the moment.

Each chapter has described a whole idea and then provided you with specifics about that idea. Knowing and remembering the pieces of these ideas and how they connect can provide you with a working plan of what you might try to do at certain times when you are interacting with others.

 KIDS IN ACTION: GETTING THE BIG PICTURE

Sean is a seventh grader who is very smart. He reads, writes, and talks as if he were in high school. Although he works well on his studies alone and gets straight A's every marking period, he has difficulty participating in group projects. He doesn't mind working with other kids, but sometimes he gets very stuck on rules and details. When he sees that something might be different than he or the teacher expects it to be, he spends a lot of time reminding the other students about what he believes is the "right way" to do things. This makes it hard for the group to move forward and complete the assignment. The students who know Sean like having him in their group because he is so smart, but they also tend to get frustrated because he has a hard time communicating with them and usually ends up doing everything himself.

Before assigning the next group project, Sean's teacher decides to talk with him privately so that she can remind him ahead of time about what he will need to do in order to get along with the other students in his group and also get the work done. She explains to him that he needs to understand that the Big Picture about group projects is that everyone works together as a team and shares the responsibilities so that the work gets done. She also lets him know that he should not be so concerned about *how* the work is getting done or who is doing it.

Sean's teacher decides to give him a checklist so that he can remember all the skills he needs to be a cooperative member of his group. It includes all of the topics that help kids put together the whole of a situation just like we have discussed in this book:

- Emotions and feelings
- Self-control
- Perspective taking
- Communication/conversation
- Relationships
- Getting along with others

The teacher reminds Sean that he must attend to all of these pieces in order for him to work in the group the way that the other students expect him too.

She explains that using this checklist is a way for him to "self-monitor" or check in with himself periodically, and see if he is doing what he is supposed to so that he can change his behavior if he needs to.

Putting It All Together ...

Using information that you already know (like the steps for how to do something) and applying it right in the moment is an important part of thinking about the Big Picture. When you can do this, you will be able to plan ahead and be better prepared for what is happening around you. It will also help you understand how your thoughts, feelings, and behaviors are contributing to the situation. Being able to think about "thinking," keeping yourself organized, and planning ahead are necessary skills in social problem solving.

You have worked hard on all these things. Now this last chapter will provide you with further information about how to put it all together.

Planning, Organizing, and Prioritizing

You always need to plan, organize, and prioritize when you are in school so that you can complete your homework assignments and long-term projects. You should be able to do these things in your social life as well.

For example, you can manage your "free time" when you are not in school in a similar way, so that you can participate in activities that you enjoy and be with other people that are important to you.

Planning

Planning means that you are developing ideas in your head and getting prepared to move forward with them.

You might "plan" or choose an activity you want to do or a project you want to complete so that you can get prepared ahead of time. For example, you must plan ahead if you want to be with a friend, otherwise he may be busy when you want to see him.

Suppose there is a movie you would really like to see and you want to go with your best friend. The weekend is a great time to go to the movies with a friend. But if you wait until it is Friday, Saturday, or Sunday to call someone to see if they can go with you, there is a strong possibility that they already have plans and will not be available to spend time with you.

Using tools like a calendar or a planner can help you remember to plan ahead to make all the arrangements you need to in order to spend time with your friends.

Organizing

After you have developed a plan for what you want to accomplish, you need to organize all the thoughts and ideas you have that relate to what you want to do.

You can organize by making lists in your head or writing them down on paper. Your lists should cover things like time, tools/equipment, money, or help you might need. You may also want to consider asking if a friend would be interested in doing it with you. Having someone join you can make things easier and more fun.

Let's continue with the example from before. It's Monday. You decide that you want to go to see a movie with your best friend on Saturday during the day and you have planned ahead. Now, you can put a list together of all the steps you need to take so that you can make sure your plans actually happen. Your list will probably include things like:

- Phoning your friend and asking if he would like to go with you
- Finding out where and when the movie is playing
- Asking your parents or your friend's parents for a ride if you need it
- Finding out how much money you need to pay for a ticket

Planning and organizing will help make it easier for you to complete things and tasks. It will also allow others to help you better (e.g., your parents will have enough notice to plan to drive you to the movies if that is what you want to do). This shows that you are thinking about others.

Prioritizing

Prioritizing involves making decisions about which items on your list are the most important and need to be completed first.

You might number the items on the list that you made on paper to show how important you think each item is. That will also show you where you should begin.

Continuing on with the movie example, you might think about which item, or items, on the list are the most important. These are the ones you should do first. The first item on the list is "Phoning your friend to see if they are available and want to go to the movies with you."

This was chosen as number one because it is the most important. If your friend can't or doesn't want to go with you, you will have to find someone else, go alone, or not go at all. These are options you will have to consider after finding out if what you want to do is possible.

When you prioritize, you are better able to manage many things at once, and it will be easier for you to get help if you need it.

Social Problem Solving and Big Picture Thinking

Now that you have been through all the chapters in this book, you probably have a list in your head of the things that were discussed: emotions, self-control, perspective taking, communication, relationships, and interactions. These are the individual parts, but remember that you should view social situations as a whole, and not in parts. This is the way that most social interactions and problem solving happens.

When you are applying Big Picture Thinking to your own life experiences, you can and should:

1. Observe first, act second.
2. Pretend your eyes are a camera and take a clear picture of what is going on around you.
3. Notice **what** is happening in the moment. Look carefully at the surroundings, where you are and what you are doing.
4. Take a good look at the **people** in the situation.
5. Try to understand what the people involved are feeling and thinking.
6. Try to understand what **you** are feeling and thinking.
7. Be a good communicator.
8. Enjoy the relationships and the experiences that you have with other people.

Big Picture Thinking

Understanding the Big Picture is all about thinking about situations as a whole rather than parts.

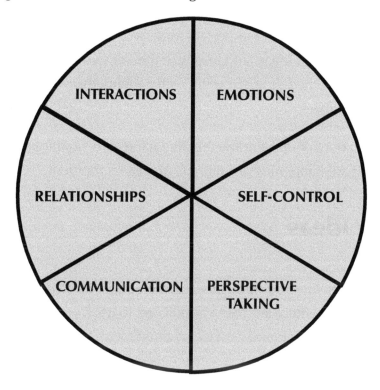

Remembering to put all the pieces together can help us to be more successful in social situations.

 KIDS IN ACTION REVIEW

At the beginning of this chapter, you read about Sean who was having a lot of difficulty working with other students in a group. Because he seemed to be very focused on the "specifics" when working on a group project, it may be helpful for him to sit down and review Big Picture Thinking so that he can have a better idea about how to fit those smaller details into a whole and arrive at a better outcome.

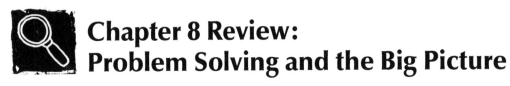

Chapter 8 Review:
Problem Solving and the Big Picture

Planning, organizing, and prioritizing are important aspects of accomplishing goals. You need to plan ahead, organize your thoughts and ideas, and prioritize the steps you have to take for any project, big or small, including things like scheduling an outing with a friend, throwing a party, or even when you join in a conversation with others.

Social problem solving is about understanding the Big Picture of a situation and not just getting stuck on the smaller details that are happening around you at a given moment.

 Practice Ideas

1. **Use Graphic Organizers.** Get your thoughts down on paper to help you plan, organize, prioritize, and solve problems. There are many good ways to track your thoughts and help you understand the Big Picture of a problem, activity, or assignment. You may have seen some of these visual organization tools before, since many teachers use them in the classroom when they are presenting a new topic or to help students with writing assignments. They are also helpful for taking notes in class or doing "research" assignments. A few different graphic organizers are described below, with some examples. You can find blank copies of all of them in the Appendix of this book on pages A18-A20.

    Spider Map – A good way to track your thoughts is to use a semantic map or "spider diagram." The "big" idea goes in the middle as the body of the spider and the related ideas have lines reaching the middle as the spider's legs:

    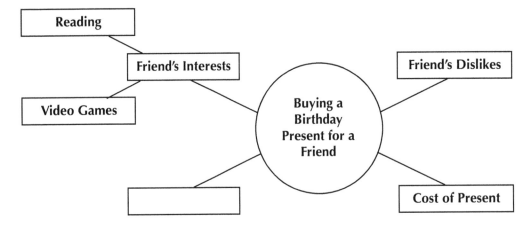

    In the example above, the body of the spider is titled "Buying a birthday present for a friend." The legs include all the things you need to consider when choosing a present. For example, the upper-left leg says "friend's interests," and the branches that follow it are examples of things that a friend might like. Those ideas will be right there on the page to help you get started when you are trying to think of what to buy. In the above case, maybe the friend might like something to do with reading or video games.

Describing Wheel – Use a "describing wheel" to help you organize your thoughts on paper. This can be for an activity you are planning, an assignment you are working on, or to look at your thoughts about a social problem you are facing.

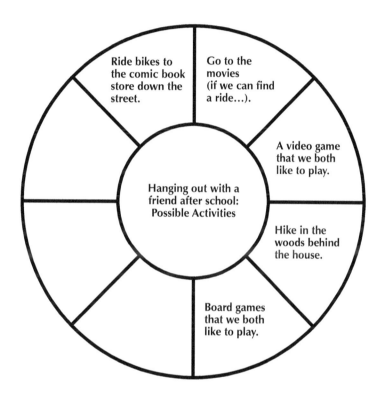

2. **Review Your Thoughts and Ideas in #1 With Someone You Trust.** The old saying "Two heads are better than one" is a helpful reminder here. Letting someone new look at your ideas will help you organize your thoughts and come up with new ideas. This is also called "getting a second opinion."

3. **Think Flexibly**. Playing games that help you stretch your mind is very helpful in keeping your thinking "flexible." Games you might play include the following:

   • **Definitions** – Play with a partner (you plus one other person) or a group. Make a list of words from the dictionary that you (and your partner) have never seen before and for which you have no idea of the correct meaning. You could also do a search on the Internet for "strange" or "difficult" words. Put each word with its correct definition on an index card and place the cards in a pile. For each round, have someone be the "moderator" and choose a card with a word and definition on it, that way they will be the only one who knows the correct meaning of the word.

Have the other player(s) guess the definition of the unknown word by writing their idea down on paper without showing or telling it to anybody. Then have the moderator read the "invented" definitions along with the correct one. The players group can vote on which meaning they think is the correct one. Give players 10 points for guessing the correct definition and 5 points for every vote their "fake" definition receives.

- **Connections** – This activity can be done alone or with two or more people. Take two seemingly random words or ideas from a dictionary or encyclopedia and see how many similarities you can find between them. For example, take the words "blanket" and "taco." Both have two syllables, both can be folded, etc. If you are playing by yourself, ask an adult to look over your list of similarities. If you are playing with a partner, review your lists together. Any items on your lists that are the same get eliminated. Players get 10 points for each of the ideas they have remaining. The one with the highest number of points is the winner.

- **Category Brainstorm** – This can be played alone or with two or more people. Pick a "category," and with a time limit, list as many words or sayings you can think of that belong to the category. You can choose easy categories like furniture or toys at first. As you get better, give yourself more of a challenge. Some ideas:

  1. Things that are yellow

  2. Words or sayings that include the word "cat" (category, "Cat in the Hat," catastrophe, etc.)

  3. Three-letter words

  4. Foods that are white

  5. Sticky things

  Give yourself a 1-minute time limit for easy categories and 2 or 3 minutes for harder ones. After your time limit is up, review your list. If you are playing alone, ask an adult to review the list with you. They can add things for you, too. If you are playing with a partner, review your lists together. Any ideas on your lists that are the same get eliminated and then give out 10 points for every idea remaining.

- **Alpha Sequence** – In this game, you will be finding three-letter sequences within words. There are two versions of the game.

  Version 1: Take one of the three letter sequences listed below, and list as many words as you can that contain that sequence. The letters do not have to be next to each other, but they need to be in order. For example, with the letter sequence "hit" you could list the following words: height, white, or hint. The letter sequence is in order, but the letters do not have to be right next to each other.

Version 2: Take one of the three letter sequences listed below and list as many words as you can that contain that sequence. The letters can be in any part of the word (beginning, middle, or end), but they MUST be in order and directly next to each other. For example, with the letter sequence "ICO," you could list the following words: "icon," "apricot," "licorice," and "unicorn." The letter sequence is within the word and in the same order.

- **ALPHA Sequence Ideas**

"ICO"	"DER"	"OXY"
"ERT"	"HIT"	"INK"
"AZI"	"PIT"	"ICE"
"ADI"	"RIO"	"ASK"
"AGE"	"UNC"	"PAR"
"ARG"	"EST"	"PRE"

- **Cross-Categories** – In the example below, you will see a grid with categories to the left of each row and letters at the top of each column. Fill in each box with a category member that begins with the letter above each of the five columns. Try to list at least one answer in every box; some boxes will have more than one correct answer.

	D	A	B	S	P
State Capitals					
Cartoon Characters					
Television Comedies					
Jobs/Professions					
Movies					

Make this game even harder by adding a 3- or 5-minute time limit to complete the grid. (See the Appendix, page A21, for more examples.)

- **Puzzles** – All kinds of puzzles are helpful for flexible thinking, jigsaw puzzles, word searches, crossword puzzles, word jumbles, etc.

- **Humor and Jokes** – In order to understand humor and jokes both visually and auditorily, you need to have a good understanding of perspective and language. You also need to be able to make smart guesses, or infer things that aren't said. Jokes and comics are funny because they "play" with language and words and also with the perspective of the "characters" involved.

Using appropriate joke books, humorous comic strips, and/or regular books is a great way to stretch your flexible thinking skills, not to mention being better prepared to tell and receive jokes verbally with friends. The following are appropriate comics for practice:

- *Calvin and Hobbes* – Bill Watterson

- *The Far Side* – Gary Larson

- *Close to Home* – John McPherson

- *Non-Sequitur* – Wiley Miller

4. **Stay Organized When Working on a Project.** Make sure you have all the necessary materials available if you are working on something that requires writing, or if you need to save work from one day to the next. Pens, pencils, erasers, paper or notebooks, and folders should be available. Color-code your folders so that you know right away where your work is the next time you need it.

5. **Practice Problem Solving.** With an adult, think of some pretend problems and solve them. Some examples are listed below for you to start with. You can also use social situations that have happened to you or others. Write each problem on an index card; keep them together because you can use them again later. Be able to give a short "main idea" statement about what the problem is and why it needs to be solved. Then think of as many ideas as possible for solutions. Even "unsuccessful solutions" should be considered. Here is a list of problems to get you started:

- A girl at your school who is a terrific athlete wants to join your school's boys football team.

- You are going to see a movie with a friend, and you both want to see something different.

- You notice that two students in your math class are always sharing answers on their homework assignments before they turn them in to the teacher.

- A friend wants to tell her parents that she is hanging out at your house on Saturday night. In reality, she is planning to go to a party with her boyfriend that her parents told her she wasn't allowed to go to.

- You are taking care of your neighbors' two cats while they are away. You go to feed the cats on the last day and notice that you left the door open to the room they are supposed to stay in. The cats got out and have knocked over and broken a very expensive vase.

- You ask a friend to borrow his favorite video game for one week. While you have it, your little sister spills milk all over it, and it stops working.

6. **Write in Your Journal.** Use your journal to write about "problems" you have encountered with others. This is helpful if you need to talk about it with a grownup or just think about it more on your own. Learning from our own experiences is also a part of the Big Picture in social situations. Looking back through this type of journal might help you answer questions such as the following:

- What kinds of problems are you having with other kids?

- Are any of the problems similar?

- Are you making the best choices for solutions?

- Are you learning from the mistakes you make or making the same mistakes?

Wow! Can you believe it? You made it all the way through this book, Congratulations! Obviously, you've done some really great work and you should be really proud of yourself. But… remember that this is only the beginning. Keep practicing and continue learning because that's what Big Picture Thinkers do.

References

American Psychiatric Association. (2000). *Diagnostic and statistical manual of mental disorders, fourth edition, text revision.* Washington, DC: Author.

Angeli, E., Wagner, J., Lawrick, E., Moore, K., Anderson, M., Soderland, L., & Brizee, A. (2010). *General format.* Retrieved from http://owl.english.purdue.edu/owl/resource/560/01/

Baron-Cohen, S. (1999). The extreme male-brain theory of autism. In H. Tager-Flusberg (Ed.), *Neurodevelopmental disorders* (pp. 401-430). Cambridge, MA: MIT Press

Baron-Cohen, S., Leslie, A. M., & Frith, U. (1985). Does the autistic child have a "theory of mind"? *Cognition, 21,* 37-46.

Buron, K. D. (2007). *A "5" is against the law! Social boundaries: Straight up!:* Shawnee Mission, KS: AAPC Publishing.

Buron, K. D., & Curtis, M. (2003). *The incredible 5-point scale: Assisting students with autism spectrum disorders in understanding social interactions and controlling their emotional responses.* Shawnee Mission, KS: AAPC Publishing.

Conway M., Anderson, J., Larsen, S., Donnelly, C., McDaniel, M., McClelland, A., Rawles, R., & Logie, R. (1994). The formation of flashbulb memories. *Memory and Cognition, 22,* 326-343.

Easterbrook J. (1959) The effect of emotion on cue utilization and the organization of behavior. *Psychological Review, 66,* 183-201.

Frith, U. (1989). Autism and "theory of mind." In C. Gillberg (Ed.), *Diagnosis and treatment of autism* (pp. 33-52). New York, NY: Plenum Press.

Goleman, D. (2006a). *Emotional intelligence.* New York, NY: Bantam-Dell.

Goleman, D. (2006b). *Social intelligence: The new science of human relationships.* New York, NY: Bantam-Dell.

Gray, C. (1994). *The new Social Story™ book: Illustrated edition.* Arlington, TX: Future Horizons.

Gray, C. (2010). *The new Social Stories™ book: 10th anniversary edition.* Arlington, TX: Future Horizons.

Happé, F. (1999). Autism: *Cognitive deficit or cognitive style? Trends in Cognitive Sciences,* 3 (6), 216-222.

Kensinger, E. (2004). Remembering emotional experiences: The contribution of valence and arousal. *Reviews in Neuroscience, 15,* 241–251.

Lahey, M. (1988). *Language disorders and language development.* New York, NY: Macmillan Publishers.

McEvoy, R., Rogers, S., & Pennington, B. (1993). Executive function and social communication deficits in young autistic children. *Journal of Child Psychology and Psychiatry, 34,* 563-578.

Myles, B. S., Trautman, M. L., & Schelvan, R. L. (2004). *The hidden curriculum: Practical solutions for understanding unstated rules in social situations.* Shawnee Mission, KS: AAPC Publishing.

Phelps-Terasaki, D., & Phelps-Gunn, T. (2007). *Test of pragmatic language: Examiner's manual* (2nd ed.). Austin, TX: Pro-Ed.

Plaisted, K., Saksida, L., Alcantara, J., & Weisblatt, E. (2003). Towards an understanding of the mechanisms of weak central coherence effects: Experiments in visual configural learning and auditory perception. In U. Frith & C. Hill (Eds.), *Autism: Mind and brain* (pp. 187-210). Oxford, UK: Oxford University Press.

Schwartz, J., & Begley, S. (2002). *The mind and the brain: Neuroplasticity and the power of mental force.* New York, NY: Regan/HarperCollins Publishers.

Wieder, S., & Greenspan, S. (2005). Can children with autism master the core deficits and become empathetic, creative and reflective? A ten to fifteen year follow-up of a subgroup of children with autism spectrum disorders (ASD) who received a comprehensive developmental, individual-difference, relationship-based (DIR) approach. *The Journal of Developmental and Learning Disorders, 9,* 39-61.

Winner, M. G. (2006). *Inside out: What makes the person with social-cognitive deficits tick?: Asperger Syndrome, high-functioning autism, nonverbal learning disabilities (NLD), pervasive developmental disorder-not otherwise specified (PDD-NOS), hyperlexia: The I LAUGH approach.* San Jose, CA: Think Social Publishing.

Winner, M. G. (2007a). *Thinking about you, thinking about me.* San Jose, CA: Think Social Publishing.

Recommended Readings

Attwood, T. (1998) *Asperger's Syndrome: A guide for parents and professionals.* London: Jessica Kingsley.

Attwood, T. (2006). *The complete guide to Asperger's Syndrome.* London: Jessica Kingsley.

Baron-Cohen, S. (1995). *Mindblindness: An essay on autism and theory of mind.* Cambridge, MA: MIT.

Baron-Cohen, S. (2003). *The essential difference: The truth about the male and female brain.* New York, NY: Basic.

Baron-Cohen, S., Tager-Flusberg, H., & Cohen, D. (2005). *Understanding other minds: Perspectives from developmental cognitive neuroscience.* Oxford, UK: Oxford University Press.

Berscheid, E., & Peplau, L. A. (1983). The emerging science of relationships. In H. H. Kelley et al. (Eds.), *Close relationships* (pp. 1-19). New York, NY: W. H. Freeman and Company.

Buron, K. D. (2006). *When my worries get too big!: A relaxation book for children who live with anxiety.* Shawnee Mission, KS: AAPC Publishing.

Cumine, V., Dunlop, J., & Stevenson, G. (1998). *Asperger Syndrome: A practical guide for teachers.* London: D. Fulton.

Dalgleish, T., & Power, M. (1999). *Handbook of cognition and emotion.* Chichester, UK: Wiley.

Davies, A. (2004). *Teaching Asperger's students social skills through acting.* Arlington, TX: Future Horizons.

Diamond, S. (2011). *Social rules for kids – The top 100 social rules kids need to succeed.* Shawnee Mission, KS: AAPC Publishing

Dowd, T., & Tierney, J. (2005). *Teaching social skills to youth: A step-by-step guide to 182 basic to complex skills plus helpful teaching techniques.* Boys Town, NE: Boys Town Press.

Dunn, M. A. (2006). *S.O.S: Social skills in the schools: A social skills program for children with pervasive developmental disorders, including high-functioning autism and Asperger Syndrome, and their typical peers.* Shawnee Mission, KS: AAPC Publishing.

Ekman, P. (1999). Facial expressions. In T. Dalgleish & M. Power (Eds.), *Handbook of cognition and emotion* (pp. 301-320). New York, NY: John Wiley & Sons Ltd.

Ekman, P. (1999). Basic emotions. In T. Dalgleish & M. Power (Eds.), *Handbook of cognition and emotion* (pp. 45-60) West Essex, UK: John Wiley & Sons Ltd.

Ekman, P. (2009). *Telling lies: Clues to deceit in the marketplace, politics, and marriage.* New York, NY: W.W. Norton.

Faherty, C., & Mesibov, G. (2000). *Asperger's: What does it mean to me? : A workbook explaining self-awareness and life lessons to the child or youth with high-functioning autism or Aspergers: Structured teaching ideas for home and school.* Arlington, TX: Future Horizons.

Frankel, F. (1996). *Good friends are hard to find: Help your child find, make, and keep friends.* Los Angeles, CA: Perspective Publishing.

Frankel, F. D., & Myatt, R. (2003.) *Children's friendship training.* New York, NY: Brunner-Routledge.

Frith, U., & Happé, F. (1994). Autism: Beyond "theory of mind." *Cognition, 50,* 115-132.

Frith, U. (1991). *Autism and Asperger Syndrome.* Cambridge, UK: Cambridge University Press.

Gerrod, P. W. (2001). *Emotions in social psychology: Essential readings.* Philadelphia, PA: Psychology Press.

Gillberg, C. (1989) *Diagnosis and treatment of autism.* New York, NY: Plenum Publishing Corp.

Glickman, N. (2009). *Cognitive-behavioral therapy for deaf and hearing persons with language and learning challenges.* New York, NY: Routledge.

Goldstein, A. (2006). *The prepare curriculum: Teaching prosocial competencies.* Champaign, IL: Research Publishing.

Grandin, T., & Barron, S. (2005). *The unwritten rules of social relationships: Decoding social mysteries through the unique perspectives of autism.* Arlington, TX: Future Horizons.

Gray, C. (1994). *Comic strip conversations.* Jenison, MI: Jenison Public Schools.

Gray, C. (1995). *Social Stories™ and comic strip conversations: Unique methods to improve social understanding.* Jenison, MI: Jenison Public Schools.

Gray, C., White, A., & McAndrew, S. (2002). *My Social Stories™ book.* London: Jessica Kingsley.

Gutstein, S. (2000). *Autism and Aspergers: Solving the relationship puzzle.* Arlington, TX: Future Horizons.

Happé, F., & Frith, U. (1996). The neuropsychology of autism. *Brain, 119,* 1377-1400.

Happé, F., & Frith, U. (2006). The weak coherence account: Detail-focused cognitive style in autism spectrum disorders. *Journal of Autism and Developmental Disorders, 36*(1), 5-25.

Hodgdon, L. A. (2006). *Visual strategies for improving communication: Practical supports for school and home.* Troy, MI: QuirkRoberts Publishing.

Howley, M., & Arnold, E. (2005). *Revealing the hidden social code: Social stories for people with autistic spectrum disorders.* London: Jessica Kingsley Publishers.

Howlin, P., Baron-Cohen, S., & Hadwin, J. (1999). *Teaching children with autism to mind-read: A practical guide for teachers and parents.* Chichester, UK: J. Wiley & Sons.

Huggins, P., Shakarian, L., & Wood Manion, D. (1998). *Helping kids handle put-downs. The ASSIST program, affective/social skills: instructional strategies and techniques.* Longmont, CO: Sopris West.

Jolliffe, T., & Baron-Cohen, S. (1999). A test of central coherence theory: Linguistic processing in high-functioning adults with autism or Asperger syndrome: Is local coherence impaired? *Cognition, 71,* 149-185.

Kelly, K., & Ramundo, P. (2006). *You mean I'm not lazy, stupid or crazy?!: The classic self-help book for adults with attention deficit disorder.* New York, NY: Scribner Publishing.

Lavoie, R. (2006). *It's so much work to be your friend: Helping the child with learning disabilities find social success*. New York, NY: Touchstone.

Leslie, A. M., & Frith, U. (1988). Autistic children's understanding of seeing, knowing and believing. *British Journal of Developmental Psychology, 6*, 315-324.

Laugeson, E. A., & Frankel, F. H. (2010). *Social skills for teenagers with developmental and Autism Spectrum Disorders: The PEERS treatment manual*. New York, NY: Routledge.

Levine, M. (1993). *All kinds of minds: A young student's book about learning abilities and learning disorders*. Cambridge, MA: Educators Publishing Service.

Levine, M. (2001). Jarvis *Clutch – social spy: Guidelines for use: Enabling children and adolescents to understand and improve their social cognition*. Cambridge, MA: Educators Publishing Service.

Levine, M. (2002). *A mind at a time*. New York, NY: Simon & Schuster.

Manasco, H. (2006). *The way to a: Empowering children with autism spectrum disorders and other neurological disorders to monitor and replace aggression and tantrum behavior*. Shawnee Mission, KS: AAPC Publishing.

Matthews, J., & Williams, J. (2000). *The self-help guide for special kids and their parents*. London: Jessica Kingsley Publishers.

Mazza, N. (2003). *Poetry therapy: Theory and practice*. New York, NY: Brunner-Routledge.

McCloskey, G., Perkins, L. A., & Van Divner, B. (2009). *Assessment and intervention for executive function difficulties*. New York, NY: Routledge.

Moyes, R. A. (2001). *Incorporating social goals in the classroom: A guide for teachers and parents of children with high-functioning autism and Asperger Syndrome*. London: Jessica Kingsley Publishers.

Moyes, R. A. (2002). *Addressing the challenging behavior of children with high functioning autism/ Asperger Syndrome in the classroom: A guide for teachers and parents*. London: Jessica Kingsley Publishers.

Niedenthal, P., Krauth-Gruber, S., & Ric, F. (2006). *Psychology of emotion: Interpersonal, experiential, and cognitive approaches*. New York, NY: Psychology Press.

Notbohm, E., & Zysk, V. (2004). *1001 great ideas for teaching and raising children with autism spectrum disorders*. Arlington, TX: Future Horizons.

Nowicki, S., & Duke, M. (1992). *Helping the child who doesn't fit in*. Atlanta, GA: Peachtree Publishers.

O'Rourke, K., & Worzbyt, J. C. (1996). *Support groups for children*. New York, NY: Routledge.

Plutchik, R., & Conte, H. R. (1997). *Circumplex models of personality and emotions*. Washington, DC: American Psychological Association.

Plutchik, R., & Kellerman, H. (1980). Emotion: Theory, research and experience. *Theories of Emotion, Vol.1* (pp. 3-33). New York, NY: Academic.

Plutchik, R., & Plutchik, R. (2003). *Emotions and life: Perspectives from psychology, biology, and evolution*. Washington, DC: American Psychological Association.

Rubin, K. H., & Thompson, A. (2003). *The friendship factor: Helping our children navigate their social world – And why it matters for their success and happiness*. New York, NY: Penguin.

Saxe, R., & Baron-Cohen, S. (2007). *Theory of mind*. Hove, UK: Psychology Press.

Schwartz, L. (1989). *Think on your feet*. Santa Barbara, CA: Learning Works.

Smith Myles, B., Trautman, M., & Schelvan, R. (2004). *The Hidden Curriculum: Practical solutions for understanding unstated rules in social situations*. Shawnee Mission, KS: AAPC Publishing.

Sodian, B., & Frith, U. (1992). Deception and sabotage in autistic, retarded and normal children. *Journal of Child Psychology and Psychiatry, 33*, 591-605.

Stuart-Hamilton, I. (2004). *An Asperger dictionary of everyday expressions*. London: Jessica Kingsley.

Tager-Flusberg, H. (2000). Language and understanding minds: Connections in autism. In S. Baron-Cohen, H. Tager-Flusberg, & D. Cohen (Eds.), *Understanding other minds: Perspectives from autism and developmental cognitive neuroscience*. Oxford, UK: Oxford University Press.

Weber, A., & Craig H. (2005). *Clinical applications of drama therapy in child and adolescent treatment*. New York, NY: Brunner-Routledge.

Wiig, E. H., & Secord, W. (1989). *Test of Language Competence*. San Antonio, TX: Psychological Press.

Williams, M., & Shellenberger, S. (1996). *An introduction to how does your engine run?: The Alert Program for self-regulation*. Albuquerque, NM: TherapyWorks.

Williams, M., & Shellenberger, S. (1996). *How does your engine run?: A leader's guide to the Alert Program for self-regulation*. Albuquerque, NM: TherapyWorks.

Winner, M. G. (2007b). *Sticker strategies: Practical strategies to encourage social thinking and organization*. San Jose, CA: Think Social Publishing.

Winner, M. G., & Crooke, P. (2009). *Socially curious and curiously social: A social thinking guidebook for teens & young adults with Asperger's, ADHD, PDD-NOS, NVLD, or other murky undiagnosed social learning issues*. San Jose, CA: Think Social Publishing.

Winner, M. G., Crooke P., & Knopp, K. (2008). *You are a social detective!: explaining social thinking to kids*. San Jose, CA: Think Social Publishing.

Wolfberg, P. J. (2009). *Play and imagination in children with autism*. New York, NY: Teachers College.

Zins, J. E., Elias, M. J., & Maher, C. A. (2007). *Bullying, victimization, and peer harassment: A handbook of prevention and intervention*. New York, NY: Haworth.

Appendix

Note to Teachers and Parents: Although this book is written for young people, it is most effective when read or reviewed with an adult. As you partner with the student to support his or her understanding of the material and the practice exercises, you will also need to assist with dissemination of the materials here in this appendix.

It is suggested that you help determine what Appendix materials will be helpful for the student and prepare them (make copies or introduce verbally) as the student progresses through the book. This is particularly important for the Big Picture Thinking Checklist (A1), as it could and should be referred to throughout the reading of the book.

Big Picture Thinking Checklist

This Big Picture Thinking Checklist can be used in the following ways:

- It can be used **before** a student goes into a social situation so that he or she can be "primed" to think about Big Picture clues.

- It can be used **following** a situation as a review to "check in" and see if the student has remembered to think about Big Picture clues. When used in this way as a "post-social examination or dissection," you and the student should be able to see where breakdowns in big picture thinking have occurred, which will allow for better prompting for next time.

You can alter the language and questions in the checklist in order to accommodate past or present tense depending on when you might be reviewing it with the student.

The main idea is to be thinking about the areas that were discussed in each chapter of this book – emotions, self-control, perspective, communication, relationships – and apply them to a particular situation.

Big Picture Thinking Checklist

Place Clues – Thinking about the **physical environment** around you.	
What kind of place is this?	
Have you ever been here before?	
What is going on around you?	
What kind of behavior is expected at the place you are in?	
People Clues – Thinking about the **people** who are around you.	
Who is with you, around you, or near you?	
How well do you know the people you are with? Or the people that are near you?	
Can you tell what they are thinking about?	
What is their current mood? What do you think they might be feeling?	
What is your mood? What do you think you are feeling?	
Do you think that you are feeling the same thing as the other people you are with? Or are they feeling something different?	
Face-to-Face Clues – Thinking about the nonverbal clues that are displayed by others.	
Check their nonverbal cues:	
Body language	
Physical proximity (How close or far away from you are they?)	
Gestures	
Facial expressions	
Eye gaze (where are they looking?)	
Tone of Voice	
Check their physical appearance:	
Clothes	
Hair	
Skin color	
Age	
Height	
Weight	
Word Clues – Thinking about what is being said.	
What are the other people around you saying?	
Are they talking with you or to other people?	
Do their words match what you think they might be feeling?	
Do they mean what they are saying?	
Are you involved in the conversation?	
Are you choosing words that are appropriate for where you are and who you are with?	

Feeling Thermometer

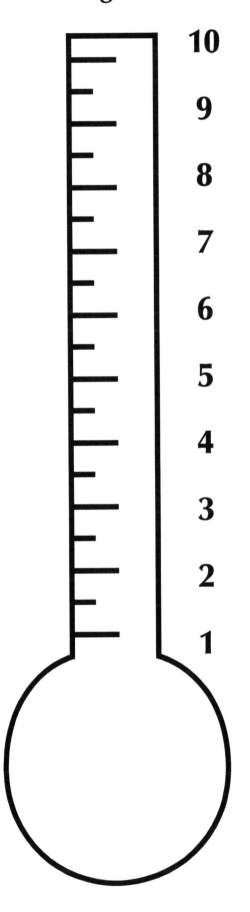

10
9
8
7
6
5
4
3
2
1

Incredible 5-Point Scale

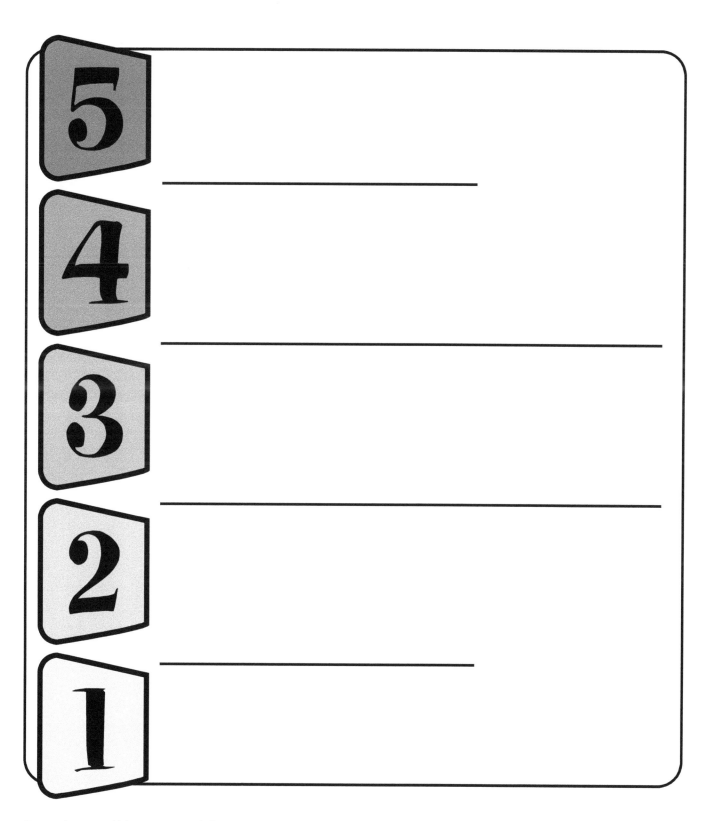

From *The Incredible 5-Point Scale* by Kari Dunn Buron and Mitzi Curtis, 2003, Shawnee Mission, KS: AAPC Publishing. Reprinted with permission.

Emotion/Behavior Tracking Worksheet

Situation	Emotion	What It Felt Like	What It Looked Like	Did I Express Myself to Others Appropriately?

5-Point Scale for Emotions

Name: _____ My _____ Scale

Rating	Looks/Sounds like	Feels like	Safe people can help/ I can try to
5			
4			
3			
2			
1			

From *The Incredible 5-Point Scale* by Kari Dunn Buron and Mitzi Curtis, 2003, Shawnee Mission, KS: AAPC Publishing. Reprinted with permission.

A "5" Could Make Me Lose Control Worksheet
Fill in you own stress scale.

Level	Person, place or thing	Makes me feel like this:
5		This could make me lose control!!!!
4		This can *really* upset me.
3		This can make me feel nervous.
2		This sometimes bothers me.
1		This never bothers me.

From *A "5" Cold Make Me Lose Control!* by Kari Dunn Buron, 2007, Shawnee Mission, KS: AAPC Publishing. Reprinted with permission.

Helpers Worksheet for Calming Strategies

Calming Strategy I tried	Did It Help Me?	When Can I Use It?
Yoga	Yes, I felt very relaxed after.	This strategy is most appropriate for home where I can be alone and relax.
Counting backward from 10-1	Yes, it helped me focus on my body and feelings instead of the things around me.	Any time I need to because I can do it in my head.

Voice Scale

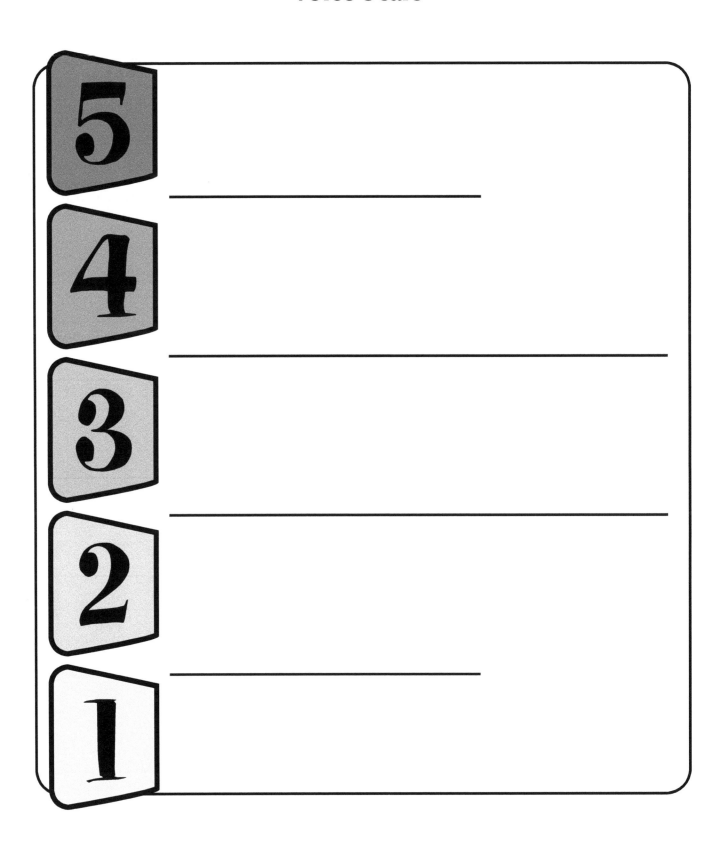

From *The Incredible 5-Point Scale* by Kari Dunn Buron and Mitzi Curtis, 2003, Shawnee Mission, KS: AAPC Publishing. Reprinted with permission.

Big Picture Communication Role-Play

Location	Person	Purpose	Topic
Library	Librarian	Asking for help	"I think I need some help finding a book for my book report."

Friends Roster

Name:	**Nickname:**
Address:	**Birthday:**
Home phone:	**Cell phone:**
Email:	**Parents:**
Other family:	
Interests:	**Friends you have in common:**
Things you enjoy doing together:	
Other information:	

Self-Monitoring "Unfriendly Behaviors" Worksheet

Unfriendly Behavior	How It Makes Others Feel	What Can I Do to Make a Change?

Self-Monitoring "Friendly Behaviors" Worksheet

Friendly Behavior	How It Makes Others Feel	What Can I Do to Make a Change?

Relationship Pyramid Worksheet

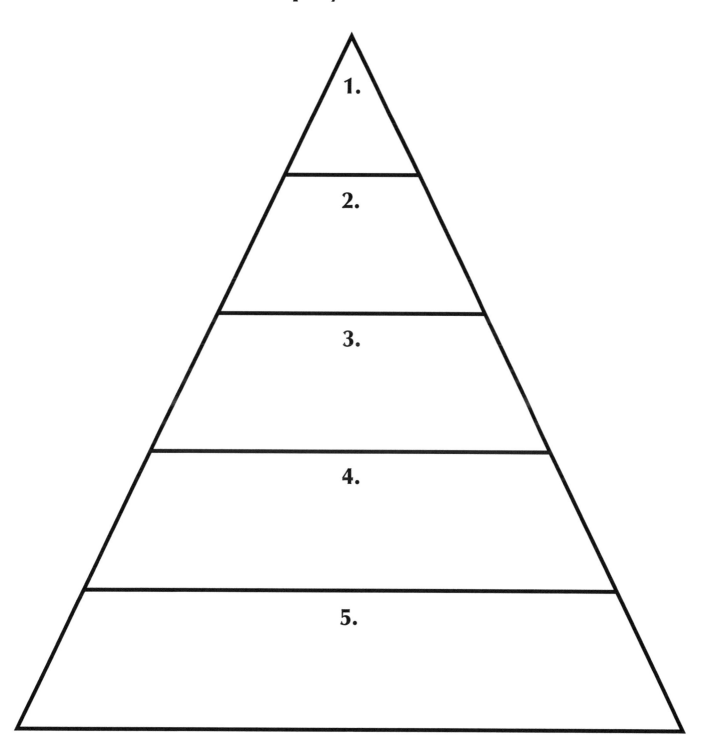

1.

2.

3.

4.

5.

"Walking in the Positive" Worksheet

What Is/Was the Situation?	How Are/Were You Feeling?	What Are/Were You Thinking?	Change Your Negative Thoughts to Positive Thoughts

Constructive Arguments Worksheet

Did I ...	Remember to be critical of ideas and not people?	Let everyone have a chance to share their thoughts?	Listen attentively to the other person's ideas?	Focus on making the best possible decision for everyone?	Generate multiple solutions to the problem and reach an appropriate agreement?
Role-Play #1					

Graphic Organizers: Spider Map

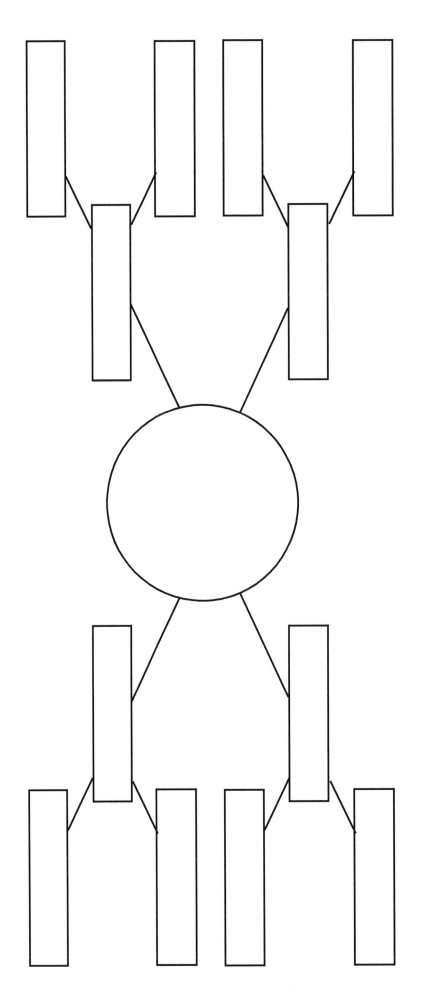

Graphic Organizers: Describing Wheel

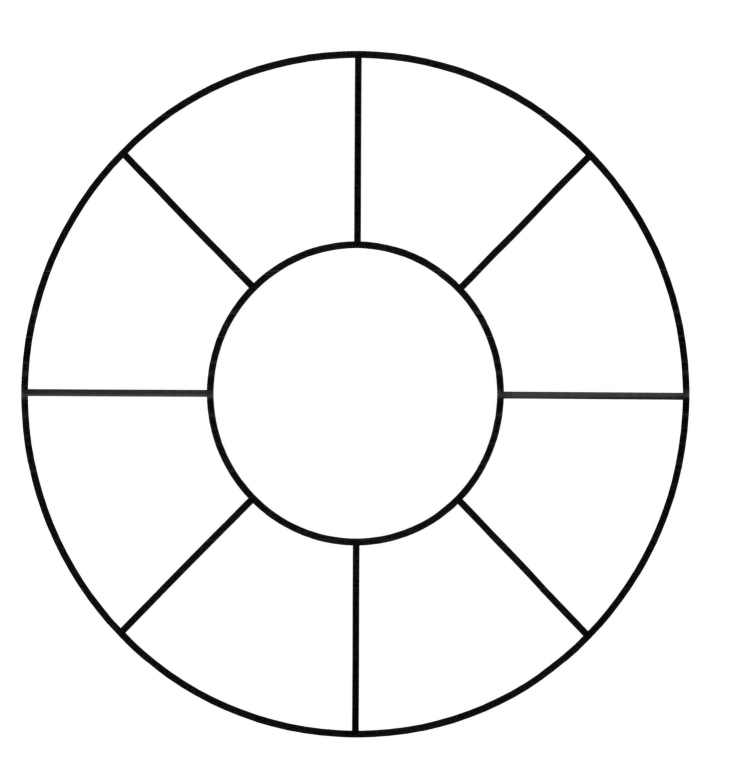

Venn Diagram for Comparing and Contrasting

Cross-Categories

	G	R	T	W	M
States					
Sports					
School Subjects					
Fruit					
Jungle Animals					

	A	E	I	O	U
Things in the Kitchen					
Sea Animals					
Vacation Spots					
Parts of a Newspaper					
Things at the Circus					

Games for Reinforcement of Social-Communication Skills

The board game ideas listed below are sorted by "category;" however, many of them fit into more than one category. Some of those that are listed are "adult" party games, but there are also "junior" versions, and I have found it easy to sort through the clue cards ahead of time in order to make sure that topics are age-appropriate.

Parents and Professionals: Review the following games ahead of time, so that you can learn how to play and decide if they are relevant to what you are attempting to help reinforce.

Games reinforce many of the social skills that have been introduced in this book, and in many social skills groups. They help support …

- Language skills – word retrieval, language formulation and organization, narrative construction, auditory working memory, sequencing
- Perspective taking skills and knowing your friends
- Team/cooperative skills
- Critical thinking/flexible thinking
- Dealing with "stress" from timed responses
- Good sportsmanship

Expressive Language/Word Retrieval

- Taboo/Taboo Jr.
- Outburst/Outburst Jr.
- Wordplay
- Twenty Questions
- Password
- Blurt
- Frazzled
- Family Feud
- Pictionary Jr.
- Word Yahtzee
- Who, What Where Jr.
- Buzzword/Buzzword, Jr.
- Perfect Sense
- Malarkey
- Balderdash
- Know It or Blow It

- Scattergories/Scattergories Jr./Scattergories Card Game
- Don't Say it
- Last Word

Memory Skills – Visual, Auditory, and Otherwise

- Concentration
- Memory
- Any game that plays "sound patterns" like Simon, Uno Blitzo, Rubiks Revenge
- I Spy Books/game

Critical Thinking Skills/Perspective-Taking Skills

- Tri-bond/Tri-bond for Kids
- 3 for Me
- Apples to Apples
- Trivial Pursuit – Children's Edition
- Mastermind
- Clue/Clue Jr. – or any other game with a similar format
- Imaginiff
- Tattletale
- Headbandz
- Guesstures
- Charades for Kids/Best of Charades for kids
- Cranium Cadoo and other Cranium Games
- True Colors
- Fib or Not

Auditory Processing/Sequencing

- Guess Who
- Sequence
- Sort It Out

Spelling/Phonemic Awareness/Vocabulary Building

- Scrabble/ Scrabble Slam
- Boggle
- Jumble Game
- Upwords
- Word Thief

Children's Literature/Bibliotherapy

Using children's books can be an effective way of communicating with your child. Books can serve as a "metaphor" for life and they can help children internalize important social skills. Books can also provide children with a clearer understanding of their own strengths and weaknesses, leaving them with a reference for the future.

There are many titles available, about all different topics – too many to list here. Searches at the library or major bookseller websites are helpful in locating the topics you may need. The following is a short list of both fiction and nonfiction titles, including some of the titles that I like to use as a starting point for certain lessons in social skills groups. Reading a book at the beginning of a session helps to introduce a concept and direct students' attention to the skills that will be targeted during the session. Similarly, reading a book at the end of a session can help to reinforce skills worked on during a session. Bibliotherapy crosses all age groups, and I have found it to be an effective tool for starting discussions, especially when students are hesitant to talk about their own experiences.

The books are listed by topic, yet many may work in more than one category. Wherever possible, I have included an age or grade range; however, I have found that using books that are at a "younger" chronological age level than the targeted audience helps to lift some of the cognitive demands and allows students to focus more directly on the content as it is related to social skills. At the same time, it is important to ensure that older students don't feel talked down to and presented with childish materials. Take a closer look prior to purchasing or borrowing from the library, to ensure you find language, pictures, and stories that are comfortable for you and your family, as well as age-appropriate for your child.

Anger

Lictenheld, T. (2003). *What are you so grumpy about?* New York, NY: Little, Brown and Company. (Grades 1-4)

Martin, J., & Marx, P. (1993). *Now everybody really hates me.* (1993). New York, NY: Harper Collins Publishers. (K-grade 2)

Shapiro, L. (1994). *The very angry day that Amy didn't have.* King of Prussia, PA: Childswork Childsplay. (Ages 4-0)

Vail, R. (2002). *Sometimes I'm bombaloo.* New York, NY: Scholastic Press. (Ages 3-7)

Verdick, E., & Lisovskis, M. (2003). *How to take the grrrr out of anger.* Mineappolis, MN: Free Spirit Publishing. (Ages 9-12)

Sibling/Family Issues (See Also Special Needs)

Blume, J., & Trivas, I. (2002). *The pain and the great one.* New York, NY: Atheneum for Young Readers. (Ages 4-8)

Crist, J. J., Verdick, E., & Mark, S. (2010). *Siblings: you're stuck with each other, so stick together.* Minneapolis, MN: Free Spirit Publishing. (Grades 5-8)

Teasing/Bullying

Best, C. (2009). *Shrinking violet.* New York, NY: Pocket Books/MTV. (Young adult)

Burnett, K. G., & Barrows, L. (2000). *Simon's hook: A story about teases and put-downs.* Roseville, CA: GR Publishers. (Grades 1-4)

Bosch, C. W., & Strecker, R. (1988). *Bully on the bus.* Seattle, WA: Parenting Press. (Grades 2-5)

Clements, A. (2001). *Jake Drake, bully buster.* New York, NY: Aladdin Library. (Grades 2-4)

Cohen-Posey, K. (1995). *How to handle bullies, teasers and other meanies.* Highland City, FL: Rainbow Books Inc. (Grades 4-6)

Cook, J. (2009) *Bully B.E.A.N.S.* Chattanooga, TN: National Center for Youth Issues. (Ages 4-8)

Cosby, B., & Honeywood, P. (2003). *The meanest thing to say.* New York, NY: Scholastic, Inc. (Grades K-3)

DePaola, T. (1995). *Oliver Button is a sissy.* San Diego, CA: Harcourt Brace Jovanovich. (Ages 4-8)

DePaola, T. (2003). *Meet the Barkers: Morgan and Moffat go to school.* New York, NY: Puffin. (Ages 4-7)

Hammerseng, K., & Garbot, D. (1996). *Telling isn't tattling.* Seattle, WA: Parenting Press. (Ages 4-8)

Jackson, J. S. (2010). *Bye-Bye, bully: A kid's guide for dealing with bullies.* St. Meinrad, IN: One Caring Place. (Ages 9-12)

Lovell, P., & Catrow, D. (2002). *Stand tall, Molly Lou Melon.* New York, NY: Putnam Publishing Group. (Ages 5-8)

Ludwig, T., & Gustavson, A. (2005). *Just kidding.* Berkley, CA: Tricycle Press. (Grades 1-5)

Ludwig, T., & Marble, A. (2005). *My secret bully.* Berkley, CA: Tricycle Press. (Grades 2-5)

Ludwig, T. (2006). *Sorry!* Berkley, CA: Tricycle Press. (Grades 2-5)

Ludwig, T. (2008). *Trouble talk.* Berkley, CA: Tricycle Press. (Grades 2-4)

Ludwig, T. (2010). *Confessions of a former bully.* Berkley, CA: Tricycle Press. (Grades 3-6)

McCain, B., & Leonardo, T. (2001). *Nobody knew what to do: A story about bullying.* Morton Grove, IL: Albert Whitman & Company. (Ages 4-8)

McLeod, S. (2007). *Hot issues, cool choices: Facing bullies, peer pressure, popularity, and put-downs.* Amherst, NY: Prometheus Books. (Ages 9-12)

Moss, M. (1999). *Amelia takes command.* Middleton, WI: Pleasant Company Publications. (Grades 3-5)

Moss, P., & Lyon, L. (2008). *Say something.* Gardiner, MD: Tilbury House Publishers. (Grades K-5)

O'Neill, A., & Huliska-Beith, L. (2006). *The recess queen.* Gosford, NSW: Scholastic. (Ages 5-8)

Polacco, P. (2001). *Thank you Mr. Falker.* New York, NY: Philomel Books. (Ages 5 and up)

Romain, T. (1998). *Cliques, phonies and other baloney.* Minneapolis, MN: Free Spirit Publishing. (Grades 3-8)

Romain, T., & Verdick, E. (2000). *Bullies are a pain in the brain.* New York, NY: Scholastic, Inc. (Grades 3-7)

Schraff, A. (2007). *The bully (Bluford High Series #5), Book 5.* New York, NY: Scholastic, Inc. (Young adult)

Thomas, P. (2000). *Stop picking on me: A first look at bullying.* Hauppauge, NY: Barrons Educational Series. (Ages 4-7)

Webster-Doyle, T. (1999). *Why is everybody picking on me: Guide to handling bullies.* Weatherhill, NY: Weatherhill. (Ages 8-14)

Friendship

Carlson, N. (1997). *How to lose all your friends.* New York, NY: Puffin. (Ages 4-7)

Carter, M., & Santomauro, J. (2010). *Friendly facts: A fun, interactive resource to help children explore the complexities of friends and friendship.* Shawnee Mission, KS: AAPC Publishing. (Ages 7-11)

Henkes, K. (1988). *Chester's way.* Hong Kong: South China Publishing Company. (Ages 3-8)

Krasny, L., & Brown, M. (2001). *How to be a friend: A guide to making friends and keeping them.* Boston, MA: Little Brown & Company. (Ages 4-8)

Wescott, N. (1996). *The care and keeping of friends (American Girl Library).* Middleton, WI: Pleasant Company Publications. (Ages 9-12)

Murrell, D. (2001). *Tobin learns to make friends.* Arlington, TX: Future Horizons. (Ages 4-8)

Murrell, D. (2007). *Friends learn about Tobin.* Arlington, TX: Future Horizons. (Ages 4-8)

Espeland, P., & Verdick, E. (2006). *Making choices and making friends: The social competencies assets (Adding Assets).* Minneapolis, MN: Free Spirit Publishing. (Ages 9-12)

Fox, A. (2009). *Real friends vs. the other kind (Middle School Confidential).* Minneapolis, MN: Free Spirit Publishing. (Grades 5-8)

Getting Along/Sharing/Conflict Resolution

Criswell, P. K., & Martini, A. (2003). *A smart girl's guide to friendship troubles.* Middleton, WI: American Girl Publishing, Inc. (Ages 9-12)

Packer, A. (2004). *The how rude! Handbook of friendship & dating manners for teens: Surviving the social scene.* Minneapolis, MN: Free Spirit Publishing. (Young adult)

Feelings/Self-Esteem

Christ, J. (2004). *What to do when you're scared and worried: A guide for kids.* Minneapolis, MN: Free Spirit Publishing. (Grades 5-8)

Espeland, P., & Verdick, E. (2005). *Proud to be you: The positive identity assets.* Minneapolis, MN: Free Spirit Publishing. (Ages 9-12)

Fox, A. (2008). *Be confident in who you are (Middle School Confidential Series).* Minneapolis, MN: Free Spirit Publishing. (Grades 5-8)

Goldblatt, R. (2004). *The boy who didn't want to be sad.* Washington DC: Magination Press. (Ages 4-8)

Henkes, K. (2000). *Wemberly worried.* New York, NY: Greenwillow Books. (Ages 9-12)

Kaufman, G. (1999). *Stick up for yourself: Every kid's guide to personal power and self-esteem.* Minneapolis, MN: Free Spirit Publishing. (Ages 9-12)

McCloud, C., & Messing, D. (2009). *Have you filled a bucket today? A guide to daily happiness for kids.* Northville, MI: Ferne. (Ages 4-8)

Petty, K., & Firmin, C. (1992). *Feeling left out.* London: Bracken. (Ages 4-8)

Romain, T., & Verdick, E. (2000). *Stress can really get on your nerves!* Minneapolis, MN: Free Spirit Publishing. (Ages 9-12)

Viorst, J. (1972). *Alexander and the terrible, horrible, no good, very bad day.* New York, NY: Atheneum Books. (Ages 5-8)

Sportsmanship

Giff, P. R. (1988). *Ronald Morgan goes to bat.* New York, NY: Puffin Books. (Grades K-3)

Welton, J. (2005). *Adam's alternative sports day: An Asperger story.* London: Jessica Kingsley. (Ages 9-12)

School Issues

Espeland, P., & Verdick, E. (2007). *See you later, procrastinator! (Get It Done)* Minneapolis, MN: Free Spirit Publishing. (Young adult)

Fox, J. S. (2006). *Get organized without losing it.* Minneapolis, MN: Free Spirit Publishing. (Grades 3-8)

Levine, M. (1990). *Keeping a head in school: A student's book about learning abilities and learning disorders.* Cambridge, MA: Educators Publishing Service. (Young adult)

Romain, T. (1997). *How to do homework without throwing up.* Minneapolis, MN: Free Spirit Publishing. (Grades 3-8)

Schumm. J. S. (2001). *School power: Study skill strategies for succeeding in school.* Minneapolis, MN: Free Spirit Publishing. (Young adult)

Manners

Cook, J. (2006). *My mouth is a volcano.* Chattanooga, TN: National Center for Youth Issues. (Ages 4-8)

Cook, J. (2007). *Personal space camp.* Chattanooga, TN: National Center for Youth Issues. (Ages 4-8)

Espeland, P., & Verdick, E. (2007). *Dude that's tude! (Get some manners).* Minneapolis, MN: Free Spirit Publishing. (Young adult)

Packer, A. (1997). *The how rude! Handbook of school manners for teens: Civility in the hallowed halls.* Minneapolis, MN: Free Spirit Publishing. (Young adult)

Verdick, E. (2010). *Don't behave like you live in a cave (Laugh and Learn).* Minneapolis, MN: Free Spirit Publishing. (Grades 4-8)

Special Needs/Differently Abled (For Children With Challenges and Their Siblings)

Bishop, B. (2003). *My friend with autism.* Arlington, TX: Future Horizons. (Ages 9-12)

Gagnon, E., & Smith Myles, B. (1999). *This is Asperger Syndrome.* Shawnee Mission, KS: AAPC Publishing. (Ages 9-12)

Hoopman, K. (2001). *Blue bottle mystery: An Asperger's adventure.* London: Jessica Kingsley Publishers. (Grades 3-5)

Hoopman, K. (2001). *Of mice and aliens: An Asperger's adventure.* London: Jessica Kingsley Publishers. (Grades 3-5)

Jackson, L., & Attwood, T. (2002). *Freaks, geeks and Asperger's Syndrome: A users guide to adolescence.* London: Jessica Kingsley Publishers. (Young adult)

Jessum, J. E. (2010). *Diary of a social detective – Real-life tales of mystery, intrigue and interpersonal adventure.* Shawnee Mission, KS: AAPC Publishing. (Ages 7-12)

Kavan, B. (2010). *Trainman: Gaining acceptance ... and friends ... through special interests.* Shawnee Mission, KS: AAPC Publishing. (Ages 4-10)

Levine, M. (1993). *All kinds of minds: A young student's book about learning abilities and learning disorders.* Cambridge, MA: Educators Publishing Service. (Ages 6 and up)

Levine, M. (2001). *Jarvis Clutch – Social spy.* Cambridge, MA: Educators Publishing Service. (Ages 9 and up)

Moss, H. (2010). *Middle school: The stuff nobody tells you about – A teenage girl with high-functioning Autism shares her experiences.* Shawnee Mission, KS: AAPC Publishing. (Grade 5 and up)

Niner H. (2003). *Mr. worry: A story about OCD.* Morton Grove, IL: Albert Whitman & Company. (Grades K-4)

Niner, H., & Treatner, M. (2005). *I can't stop!: A story about Tourette Syndrome.* Morton Grove, IL: Albert Whitman & Company. (Grades K-4)

Schnurr, R., & Strachan, J. (1999). *Asperger's huh? A child's perspective.* Gloucester ON, Canada: Anisor Publishing. (Ages 6-12)

Trautman, M. L. (2010). *My new school: A workbook to help students transition to a new school.* Shawnee Mission, KS: AAPC Publishing. (Ages 4-10)

Welton, J. (2003). *Can I tell you about Asperger Syndrome? A guide for friends and family.* London: Jessica Kingsley. (Ages 9-12)

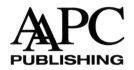

AAPC Publishing
6448 Vista Dr.
Shawnee, KS 66218
www.aapcpublishing.net